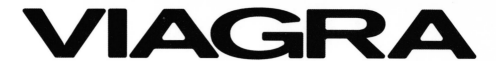

VIAGRA

(sildenafil citrate)

THE REMARKABLE STORY OF THE DISCOVERY AND LAUNCH

Larry Katzenstein
Medical Writer

Medical Editor
Eric B. Grossman, MD, FACP

Medical Director
Sexual Health Team
Pfizer Pharmaceuticals Group
Pfizer Inc.

Adjunct Associate Professor of Medicine
New York University School of Medicine
New York, New York

With illustrations by
Michael Linkinhoker and Leo Kundas

MEDICAL INFORMATION PRESS
NEW YORK

Cover design by Rob Crow
Cover photograph by Peter Tenzer
Text design by Rob Crow and Pat Walsh

Printed in Taiwan

First published in 2001   7 6 5 4 3 2 1

FOREWORD

Personal gratification in biomedical research is infrequent and is often countered by the pressures and frustrations associated with basic research. As a pharmacologist, I find it gratifying to learn that basic research can and does lead to the development of new drugs for the diagnosis, prevention, and treatment of disease. It is particularly gratifying when one's own basic research leads to the marketing of a long-awaited novel drug for the treatment of a condition that afflicts millions of people worldwide. When my colleagues and I started conducting research on the causes of erectile dysfunction (ED) in 1990, there was no effective oral treatment for ED available. Our discovery that the tiny molecule nitric oxide (NO) is the principal neurotransmitter mediating penile erection, and that the vasodilator action of NO is mediated by cyclic guanosine monophosphate (cGMP), paved the way for the development of sildenafil citrate (Viagra) as a treatment for ED.

NO is a unique signaling molecule in the body. This small gaseous molecule functions to dilate arteries and veins, prevent thrombosis and hemostasis, and inhibit vascular smooth muscle growth. NO also functions outside the cardiovascular system to slow the inflammatory process, relax nonvascular smooth muscle, and regulate learning, memory, olfaction, and autonomic activity. The antiangina drug nitroglycerin works by an NO mechanism, by undergoing conversion or metabolism to NO in vascular smooth muscle cells. Viagra enhances certain effects of NO indirectly by enhancing the actions of cGMP. I anticipate the development and marketing of many novel therapeutic strategies based on the discovery of the role of NO. Viagra represents the first successful drug in what promises to be a long and exciting list of drugs.

Viagra (sildenafil citrate): The Remarkable Story of the Discovery and Launch gives an informative and accurate account of the history of the development of Viagra and how basic research and astute clinical observations led to the marketing of one of the most novel and long-needed drugs in history. The story of Viagra should be one that is remembered as we move forward in research and development to provide society with drugs of the future.

Louis J. Ignarro, PhD
Nobel Laureate
Professor of Pharmacology
University of California
at Los Angeles

Larry Katzenstein is the former medical editor of *American Health* magazine and served for 12 years as a health writer at *Consumer Reports*. He has bachelor's and master's degrees in biology from Trinity College (Connecticut) and the University of Delaware, respectively, and a master's degree in journalism from the University of Missouri. He has earned national recognition for his medical writing, including the New York Newspaper Guild's Page One Award for Excellence in Journalism, the American College of Allergy and Immunology Media Award, and the William Harvey Award for journalistic achievement on hypertension.

PREFACE

Since its introduction in March 1998, Viagra (sildenafil citrate)—the first oral drug for treating erectile dysfunction (ED)—has received more media attention than any other drug in history. But despite (or perhaps because of) all this exposure, myths and misconceptions about both Viagra and ED abound—not only among the public but among physicians as well.

Viagra (sildenafil citrate): The Remarkable Story of the Discovery and Launch recounts Viagra's discovery in the words of the scientists involved, its evolution from antiangina drug to ED treatment, its thorough testing in large-scale clinical trials, and its blockbuster launch following Food and Drug Administration approval. The book also sets the record straight on Viagra's safety profile and, finally, it describes Viagra's impact on patients, their partners, and society.

In addition to recounting the tale of the scientific discovery of Viagra, the book provides practical advice—directly from physicians who have prescribed Viagra to their patients. And because many physicians, like their patients, are still uncomfortable talking about sex, the book gives guidelines on how to initiate that conversation so that ED can be diagnosed and treated.

As of late 2000, Viagra has prompted some 10 million men in the United States and around the world to seek treatment and get results for a problem that many had lived with in silence and shame. Above all, this is the story of a drug that has made a significant difference in the lives of millions of men and their partners.

I want to thank some of the people who gave me crucially important help with this book. My thanks go first of all to several of the researchers who were involved in Viagra's discovery and development and were kind enough to describe their roles to me. I'm also grateful to the many professionals at Pfizer who sat down with me to recall those heady days. Dr. Richard Sadovsky, a primary care physician in Brooklyn, New York, helped me by describing his approach to diagnosing and treating ED. Finally, special thanks to Carolyn Rice and Jennifer Mitchell of CMD Publishing, the kind taskmasters who oversaw this book's gestation and were a pleasure to work with.

Larry Katzenstein

March 1998 US FDA approves Viagra as the first oral medication for the treatment of ED.

1997 Pfizer files a New Drug Application for Viagra with the US Food and Drug Administration (FDA). The agency gives Viagra priority review status, which is reserved for drugs that represent major advances in treatment or fulfill a significant medical need.

1994–1997 21 clinical trials on sildenafil citrate, now known as Viagra, involve nearly 4500 men with ED.

1994 Pfizer scientists detect the enzyme PDE 5 in corpus cavernosal tissue, confirming that sildenafil's mechanism of action in treating ED is by inhibiting PDE 5.

1994 Pfizer accelerates its research pace on sildenafil citrate as a treatment for ED.

Early 1994 Second pilot study on sildenafil as an ED treatment shows that a single dose is capable of enabling erections.

VIAGRA (SILDENAFIL CITRATE) TIMELINE

1989 Pfizer scientists synthesize sildenafil citrate.

1991 Two researchers at Pfizer Central Research in Sandwich, England—Peter Ellis and Nick Terrett— note that drugs capable of inhibiting phosphodi- esterase type 5 (PDE 5) might be helpful in treating erectile dysfunction (ED).

1991 Early phase 1 studies of sildenafil citrate for treating angina—single-dose studies involving healthy volunteers—yield no findings of note.

1992 Second phase 1 angina study—a multiple- dose study on healthy volunteers—reveals that erections are a side effect of using the drug.

1992 First and only phase 2 clinical trial of sildenafil citrate as a treatment for angina finds mild hemodynamic effects.

Late 1993 First pilot study on sildenafil citrate as a treatment for ED is carried out in Bristol, England. Men took the drug 3 times a day for a week.

CONTENTS

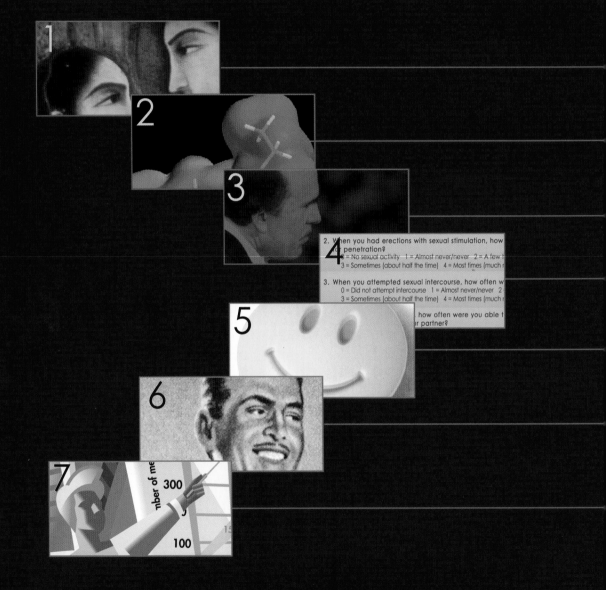

2. When you had erections with sexual stimulation, how
penetration?
0 = No sexual activity   1 = Almost never/never   2 = A few t
3 = Sometimes (about half the time)   4 = Most times (much r

3. When you attempted sexual intercourse, how often w
0 = Did not attempt intercourse   1 = Almost never/never   2
3 = Sometimes (about half the time)   4 = Most times (much r

how often were you able t
r partner?

Throughout the ages, whether in ancient India or 20th-century America, men have experienced impotence.

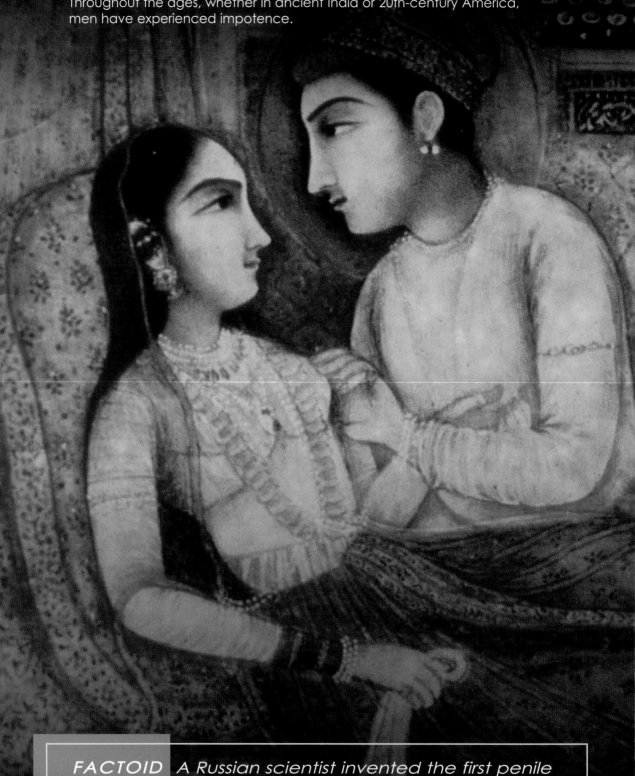

FACTOID *A Russian scientist invented the first penile implant in 1936. A piece of human rib cartilage was inserted into the penis—it didn't work.*

ERECTILE DYSFUNCTION:
A PROBLEM BOTH ANCIENT AND WIDESPREAD

1

Impotence has been a devastating problem since the beginning of recorded history. In the Bible, the Lord inflicted impotence—described as a living death—on Abimelech because he wanted to have sexual relations with Abraham's wife. "Behold thou art but a dead man, for the woman which thou has taken; for she is another man's wife" (Genesis 20:3).

A similar punishment befell King David after he impregnated the beautiful Bathsheba, wife of David's loyal soldier Uriah. David ordered Uriah into a suicidal battle so he could marry Bathsheba and declare himself the rightful father of Solomon.

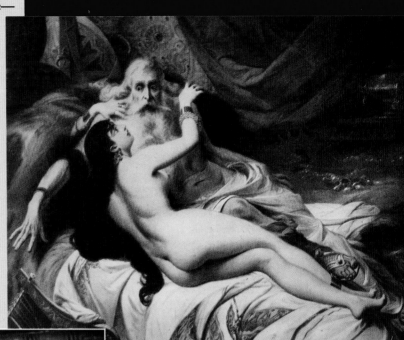

Painting by Pedro Americo of the virgin Abishag caring for the impotent King David in his old age.

Gladly I think of the days
When all my members were limber,
All except one
Those days are certainly gone,
Now all my members are stiff,
All except one

— Goethe

This ploy angered the Lord, who punished David by taking away his sword, both literally and figuratively. When his advisors presented the despondent David with the young virgin Abishag, the result was predictable: "And the damsel was very fair, and cherished the king, and ministered to him: but the king knew her not" (I Kings 1:4).

It is no surprise that impotence has long been regarded as a curse. In medieval times, it was thought to be caused by witches casting spells while acting as agents of the devil.

Literature from the 19th century also contains references to impotence (see illustration to the left).

DEMYSTIFYING THE CAUSES OF IMPOTENCE

Misperceptions about what causes impotence have persisted into this century. As recently as the 1970s, experts including Masters and Johnson insisted that virtually all cases of impotence stemmed from psychological causes.[1] But it is now known that some 80% of impotence cases are associated with physical causes such as diabetes, cardiovascular disease, or hypertension[2] (although psychological factors such as depression and anxiety are often important).

AN EXACTING TOLL ON HEALTH

Only in the past 25 years has impotence become an accepted subject for study. As researchers delved into the study of impotence, they began to realize that the toll it exacts—on both men and their relationships—is enormous. A crucial turning point occurred in 1975, when an expert committee of the World Health Organization (WHO) concluded that "problems in human sexuality are more pervasive and more important to the well-being and health of individuals in many cultures than has previously been recognized."[4]

CONDITIONS ASSOCIATED WITH ERECTILE DYSFUNCTION[3]

▶ Vascular disease

▶ Cigarette smoking

▶ Diabetes

▶ Hypertension

▶ Trauma to the spine or groin area

▶ Hormonal disorders

▶ Prostate cancer surgery

▶ Psychological problems such as anxiety and depression

▶ Many medications

▶ Alcohol or other drug abuse

IMPOTENCE GETS A NEW NAME

In 1993, the NIH Consensus Development Panel on Impotence called impotence "an important public health problem." The panel proposed that the term "impotence" be replaced by the less pejorative and more precise "erectile dysfunction" (ED) to signify "the inability to attain and/or maintain penile erection sufficient for satisfactory sexual performance."[3]

THE WORLD HEALTH ORGANIZATION DEFINES SEXUAL HEALTH[4]

Definition of sexual health: A growing body of knowledge indicates that problems in human sexuality are more pervasive and more important to the well-being and health of individuals in many cultures than has previously been recognized, and that there are important relationships between sexual ignorance and misconceptions and diverse problems of health and the quality of life. The concept of sexual health includes 3 basic elements:

1
A capacity to enjoy and control sexual and reproductive behavior in accordance with a social and personal ethic

2
Freedom from fear, shame, guilt, false beliefs, and other psychological factors inhibiting sexual response and impairing sexual relationships

3
Freedom from organic disorders, diseases, and deficiencies that interfere with sexual and reproductive functions

✓ **ED becomes increasingly prevalent with age:** 40% of men had some degree of ED at age 40; by age 50, 48% of men had some degree of ED; and by age 70, nearly 70% of men were affected.

✓ Fewer than 10% of men in the sample as a whole had complete ED, but prevalence rose sharply with age: **5% of 40-year-old men were completely impotent, compared with 15% of 70-year-olds.**

✓ **Complete ED was "significantly more prevalent" among men taking certain medications,** including antihypertensive drugs (14%), hypoglycemic drugs (26%), cardiac drugs (28%), and vasodilators (36%).

✓ **Among severely depressed men, 90% were either moderately or completely impotent.**

✓ **Cigarette smoking**—especially when combined with other health problems—**greatly increased a man's risk for ED.** For example, 56% of smokers with treated heart disease were completely impotent versus 21% of nonsmokers with treated heart disease; and 20% of smokers with treated hypertension were completely impotent versus 8.5% of nonsmokers with treated hypertension.

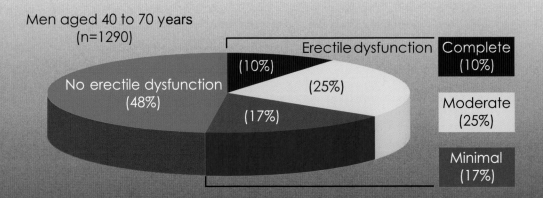

Men aged 40 to 70 years
(n=1290)

No erectile dysfunction (48%)

Erectile dysfunction

Complete (10%)

Moderate (25%)

Minimal (17%)

(10%)

(25%)

(17%)

PREVALENCE OF ED. The MMAS was a cross-sectional, random-sample survey of 1290 men 40 to 70 years old. It was conducted from 1987 to 1989 in 11 cities and towns in the Boston area. All the men filled out a sexual activity questionnaire and were interviewed by a trained technician.[5]

| CONCLUSION | MORE THAN HALF THE MEN SURVEYED HAD ED TO SOME DEGREE |

WHY SEXUAL HEALTH IS SO IMPORTANT

Men consider the ability to have erections as crucial to their sense of well-being.

Dr. Robert Salant says he has known "plenty of men" who have rejected radical prostatectomies for prostate cancer out of concern that ED would result. "This is how men think," says Dr. Salant, an associate clinical professor of urology at New York University School of Medicine in New York City. "They said they would rather take their chances with the cancer."

ED affects self-esteem and mental health.

"For many men, erectile dysfunction creates mental stress that affects their interactions with family and associates," according to the NIH consensus development report on ED.[3] "I was a person who was always full of drive, full of wanting to be involved in activities," said RT, a 48-year-old man with type 2 diabetes. "And when this part of my body started to dysfunction, it put me in kind of a depression. It was very difficult to deal with the situation where, especially in our home, things about sex were not discussed."

ED affects a man's relationship with his partner and the quality of both their lives.

At first I thought it was just a fluke," said CJ, a 46-year-old woman who was married to a man with ED. "After a while, however, I became less secure in my marriage and thought his impotence was a sign that he was no longer attracted to me. Eventually, we pretty much avoided sex, and I'm sure his sexual difficulty was one factor that led to our divorce."

"ED can precipitate a vicious cycle in which anxiety accompanies sexual activity, which in turn impedes erectile response, creating further anxiety and feelings of shame and frustration," notes Dr. Sandra Leiblum, director of the Center for Sexual and Marital Health in Piscataway, New Jersey. "Many men and women feel that it is better to avoid something that can't be taken to 'completion,' and along with sexual avoidance comes avoidance of affectionate touching. Over time, the relationship may begin to feel increasingly empty."

ED: AN ALL-TOO-COMMON PROBLEM

Gauging the extent of ED in the United States has proven notoriously difficult: The 1993 NIH consensus development report found that "appallingly little" was known on the subject.[3] Alfred Kinsey's pioneering sex surveys of the 1950s concluded that ED becomes more prevalent with age, affecting about 2% of men at age 40 and 30% at age 70.[5]

Not until the Massachusetts Male Aging Study was ED's prevalence assessed in a scientifically rigorous way. The results of the MMAS, published in 1994, revealed that the prevalence of ED far exceeded the estimates of Kinsey and other experts: a problem that to some degree affects more than half of all men aged 40 to 70.[5] Current estimates put the number of American men affected by ED at about 30 million.[3] And before Viagra (sildenafil citrate)—the first FDA-approved oral therapy for ED—was introduced in 1998, fewer than 10% of men with ED had sought treatment for their problem.[6]

SEARCHING FOR A CURE THROUGH THE AGES

Cultures throughout history have attempted to cure ED. The ancient Greeks and Egyptians concocted various anti-impotence recipes. Homer, for example, promoted the flowering jimsonweed as a possible cure. A 15th-century European text ("A Short Treatise About the People Who, Impeded by Spells, Are Unable to Have Intercourse With Their Wives") detailed how witches cause impotence (by placing "testicles of a cock under the bed," for example) and prescribed remedies for undoing witches' spells, including sprinkling the walls of one's house with dog's blood and carrying around the bile of fish.

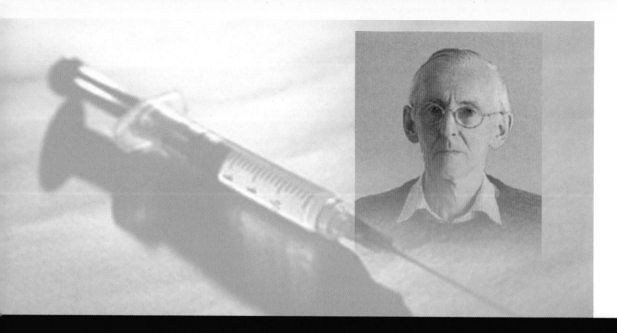

GILES BRINDLEY, MD

Real progress in treating ED did not occur until 1936, when 2 physicians—one in Russia, one in Germany—inserted human rib cartilage into the penises of impotent patients. The idea came from nature: Walruses and other mammals have permanent bonelike structures, called os penises, that guarantee potency. The inserted cartilage degraded, but these experiments ultimately led to silicone penile prostheses, which were first tried in 1973 and have proven effective.

Two important advances in ED treatment occurred in 1983. The first advance was the introduction of the vacuum constriction device. The second occurred when a British physician, Dr. Giles Brindley, demonstrated to an audience at the American Urological Association annual meeting that injecting the drug phentolamine into the penis—his, in this case—can produce an erection. This was the first evidence that ED could be successfully treated with drugs.[7] Brindley's discovery led to commercial penile injection "kits" as well as a suppository kit that inserts a drug pellet into the urethra.

FROM GILES BRINDLEY: COMMENTS ON SELF-EXPERIMENTATION

"I have a lot of slides to show, and I'm the subject in all these slides. These are drugs which when given systemically have an effect on the penis. It is in fact phentolamine that I've injected into my corpus cavernosum today, and the erection that's pushed aside by my trousers at the moment is in fact now virtually full [laughter, applause, crowd murmur]. I discovered this phenomenon last August with myself as subject, and I first tried it on a patient in November. Since then I've tried it on 15 men with erectile impotence. In 8 of them, it produced full erection; in 4 of them, though it didn't produce full erection, it made the penis stiff enough so that you couldn't bend it through a right angle. That, I reckon, permits sexual intercourse, and indeed it did so. Of these 15 men, 7 of them had sexual intercourse while under cavernosal alpha blockade, all of them for the first time in many months, most of them for the first time for years.

Until Viagra was introduced in 1998, the drugs and devices in the table to the right made up the total armamentarium of ED treatments—often effective, but shunned by the vast majority of men with ED. Prior to Viagra's introduction, only an estimated 10% of men with ED had ever tried an ED treatment.[6] Those who did start using ED treatments often stopped. In follow-up studies on intracavernosal injection therapy, many men discontinued its use after 1 or 2 years.[8-10] The breakthrough treatment for ED would have to await research that began in 1989 on a drug intended for treating angina. ●

How often can you do it? In order to satisfy the ethical committee and keep ahead of my patients, I've done it to myself. Now, I've got to look up in the table to see exactly how many times—25 times and, as you see, it still works [laughter]. **"**

Transcript of the presentation by Dr. Giles Brindley to the American Urological Association in May 1983

PRE-VIAGRA TREATMENT OPTIONS FOR ERECTILE DYSFUNCTION

YEAR INTRODUCED	NAME OF TREATMENT
1973	Penile implants
1973 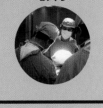	Vascular surgery to correct venous leakage
1983 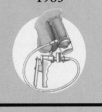	Vacuum pump
1995	Vasoactive intracavernosal pharmacotherapy
1997 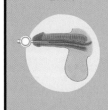	Transurethral alprostadil

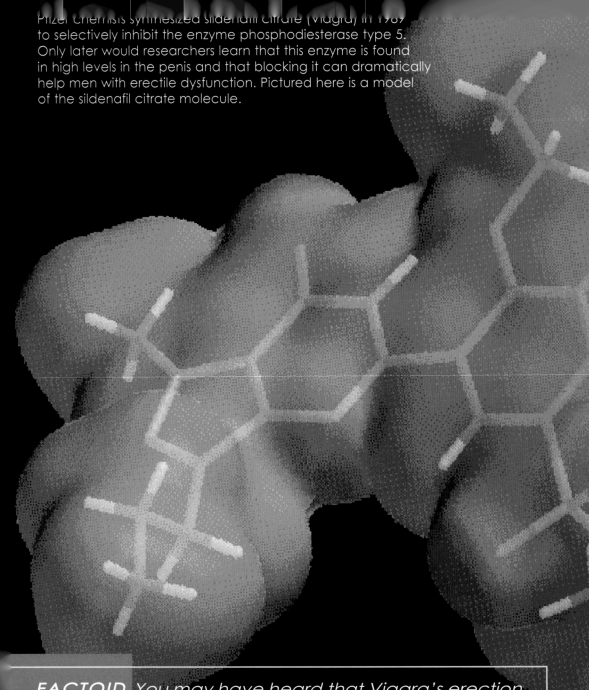

Pfizer chemists synthesized sildenafil citrate (viagra) in 1989 to selectively inhibit the enzyme phosphodiesterase type 5. Only later would researchers learn that this enzyme is found in high levels in the penis and that blocking it can dramatically help men with erectile dysfunction. Pictured here is a model of the sildenafil citrate molecule.

FACTOID *You may have heard that Viagra's erection connection was discovered in the first clinical trial for angina when patients didn't want to return their experimental pills. That's not true; in that study, Viagra was given intravenously. Later, erectile dysfunction patients in phase 3 clinical trials clamored for more Viagra as they came to the end of their study supply.*

DISCOVERING THE SILDENAFIL/ERECTION CONNECTION

Sildenafil citrate—the chemical we now know as Viagra—was not originally intended to treat erectile dysfunction (ED). Instead, it was created by scientists intent on finding a better treatment for angina.

In 1986, Pfizer researchers decided to focus on an enzyme, phosphodiesterase type 5 (PDE 5), that was present in vascular smooth muscle cells and platelets. Early in this research, they learned that inhibiting PDE 5 might produce beneficial effects: decreased vascular resistance and reduced platelet aggregation. So over the course of 3 years, Pfizer researchers synthesized and tested hundreds of compounds, and in December 1989 they found one that looked promising. It selectively targeted—and powerfully inhibited—PDE 5.

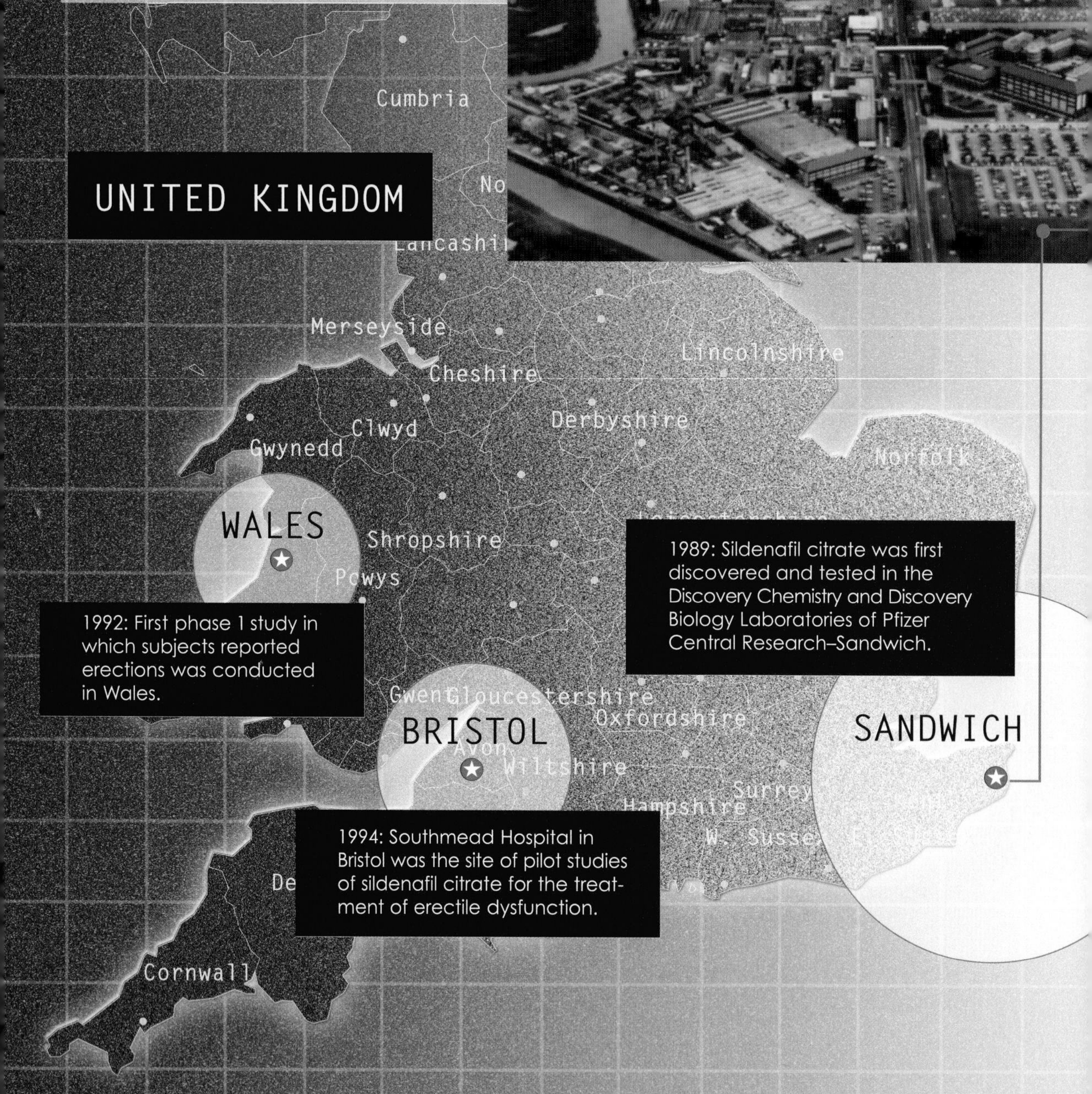

Cumbria

UNITED KINGDOM

No

Lancashi

Merseyside

Cheshire

Lincolnshire

Clwyd

Derbyshire

Gwynedd

Norfolk

WALES

Shropshire

Powys

1989: Sildenafil citrate was first discovered and tested in the Discovery Chemistry and Discovery Biology Laboratories of Pfizer Central Research–Sandwich.

1992: First phase 1 study in which subjects reported erections was conducted in Wales.

Gwen Gloucestershire

Oxfordshire

BRISTOL

SANDWICH

Avon Wiltshire

Surrey

Hampshire

W. Susse

1994: Southmead Hospital in Bristol was the site of pilot studies of sildenafil citrate for the treatment of erectile dysfunction.

De

Cornwall

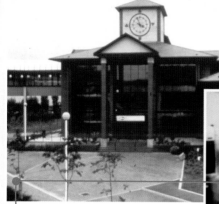

Sildenafil citrate, originally known as UK-92,480, was created in the Pfizer Discovery Chemistry Laboratory in Sandwich, England.

Theoretically, with PDE 5 inhibited, coronary arteries would dilate, thereby easing angina symptoms, and platelets would be less likely to adhere to the surface of damaged arteries where they could trigger thrombi leading to myocardial infarction. But as so often happens in scientific research, some unexpected findings arose as this new chemical entity, dubbed sildenafil citrate, traveled from lab bench to clinical trials.

TESTING SILDENAFIL AGAINST ANGINA

The earliest research on sildenafil was designed to show "proof of concept"—that the drug could cause arterial dilation and inhibit thrombus formation and therefore work against angina. Studies showed that sildenafil could relax isolated strips of artery from 2 species of animals; the drug was found to cause coronary artery dilation in dogs, rabbits, and spontaneously hypertensive rats.[6] In other studies, in which the carotid arteries of anesthesized rabbits were constricted to create a situation where thrombi formed repeatedly, sildenafil was found to inhibit thrombus formation.[6]

Clinical studies on sildenafil as an angina treatment began in 1991 in England. These phase 1 studies were designed to assess the drug's safety and determine how it affected blood pressure, electrocardiogram parameters, and other physiologic measurements. The first phase 1 study—a single-dose study involving healthy volunteers—revealed no unusual findings. In early 1992, Pfizer carried out its first multiple-dose phase 1 study of sildenafil. Healthy volunteers stayed in a hospital unit for 10 days and were given 25-, 50-, or 75-mg tablets 3 times a day.[6] Initial observations were not promising.

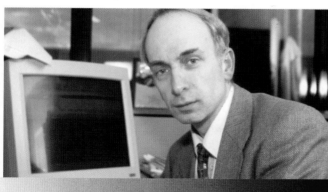

IAN OSTERLOH, MD

"A few subjects complained of vague muscle aches and backaches," recalls Dr. Ian Osterloh, the local team leader for the early sildenafil trials. But some of the men on the 2 higher doses reported another side effect as well: 5 of the 8 men taking the 75-mg dose and 3 of the 9 taking the 50-mg dose reported an increased tendency to get erections.[6]

"At the time, nobody yelled, 'Yippee, never mind the angina, what about those erections!'" Dr. Osterloh recalls.

SILDENAFIL AND HUMAN HEMODYNAMICS

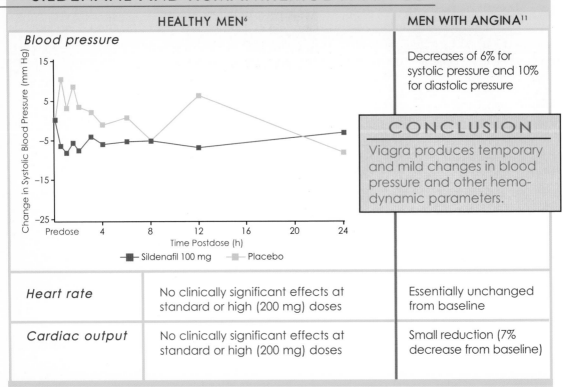

	HEALTHY MEN[6]	MEN WITH ANGINA[11]
Blood pressure	*(see graph)*	Decreases of 6% for systolic pressure and 10% for diastolic pressure
Heart rate	No clinically significant effects at standard or high (200 mg) doses	Essentially unchanged from baseline
Cardiac output	No clinically significant effects at standard or high (200 mg) doses	Small reduction (7% decrease from baseline)

CONCLUSION

Viagra produces temporary and mild changes in blood pressure and other hemodynamic parameters.

Sildenafil's effects on hemodynamics have been assessed in both healthy male volunteers and men with angina. Results, summarized in the table above, show that sildenafil produces modest, transient hemodynamic effects in both groups.

Instead, he says, "We reckoned we needed a dose of 50 mg 3 times a day for efficacy against angina and were concerned that these aches and pains would limit the dose we could give. We wondered what this would mean for the continuation of the angina program, so the erections were a bit of a side issue."

A full year would pass before this experimental heart drug's effect on erections would be studied in clinical trials. Meanwhile, researchers continued to investigate sildenafil's potential as a treatment for angina.

CHANGING DIRECTIONS: FROM TREATING ANGINA TO TREATING ED

In 1992, the first study was carried out in which sildenafil was tested on angina patients. Eight men with angina were given the drug intravenously, in doses of up to 40 mg.[11] The results are summarized in the table above.

"Sildenafil had some beneficial hemodynamic effects," Dr. Osterloh recalls. "But they were fairly mild." Several Pfizer scientists, however, urged that the drug's "erectile angle" be further explored, so the decision was made to study sildenafil specifically as a treatment for ED.

REALIZING SILDENAFIL'S POTENTIAL

Erections—sildenafil's unusual "side effect"—had not been a total surprise to Pfizer scientists who had developed the drug and knew its mechanism of action. Sildenafil's target, the enzyme PDE 5, degrades cyclic guanosine monophosphate (cGMP), a chemical that directs vascular smooth muscle cells to relax.[12] Sildenafil's action against PDE 5 therefore encouraged cGMP to accumulate; Pfizer researchers had even dubbed sildenafil "the cyclic GMP enhancer." In 1991, 2 Pfizer researchers, Drs. Peter Ellis and Nick Terrett, noted that cGMP-mediated arterial dilation not only might help relieve angina but

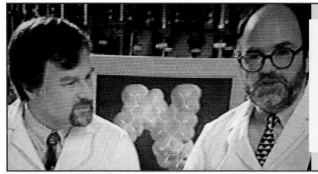

Drs. Peter Ellis and Nick Terrett in the Discovery Biology Laboratory at Pfizer Central Research in Sandwich, England. While working on potential hypertension drugs in 1991, they predicted that PDE 5 inhibitors might help in treating ED—a surmise that led to both men being named on the patent for Viagra.

also might be required for erections to occur. They speculated that sildenafil might also be useful in treating ED.

This speculation about PDE 5 inhibition bolstered the case of Pfizer scientists who lobbied for further study of the drug in treating ED. So, instead of giving up on sildenafil, Pfizer officials decided to proceed with clinical trials that would study the drug specifically as a treatment for ED.

FROM LAB BENCH TO CLINICAL TESTING

The first ED studies were designed to take advantage of emerging knowledge about how erections occur. In the early 1990s, research[13,14] at centers like the University of California at Los Angeles (UCLA) had shown that erections happen because sexual stimulation triggers nerve endings in the penis to release nitric oxide (NO),

DISCOVERING THE NITRATES CONTRAINDICATION

As part of sildenafil's early development as a treatment for angina, **Pfizer scientists realized that sildenafil (which only modestly reduces blood pressure) and organic nitrates both exert their pharmacologic effects through the same pathway.** They both raise levels of the chemical messenger cGMP, resulting in relaxation of vascular smooth muscle.

It seemed plausible that sildenafil might therefore enhance the vasodilation caused by organic nitrates, which could be a problem with an antiangina drug, since many angina patients would also be taking nitrates. So Pfizer carried out a phase 1 study to investigate such an interaction in 1992, as part of sildenafil's evaluation as an antiangina drug. In this study, which involved 12 healthy volunteers, those who received both sildenafil and sublingual glyceryl trinitrate (GTN) experienced a fourfold greater decrease in systolic blood pressure than men given a placebo and the nitrate.[15] Because of this finding of a synergistic effect between sildenafil and nitrates, **Viagra is contraindicated in men who use organic nitrates.**

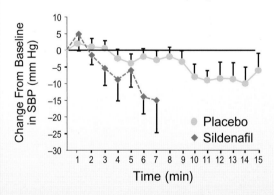

Mean maximal changes from baseline in systolic blood pressure on day 5 after sublingual GTN (500-µg tablet)[15]

During placebo treatment, 8 of 12 men completed the 15-minute GTN challenge compared with 0 of 12 men during treatment with sildenafil.

CONCLUSION

Viagra combined with an organic nitrate produces a dramatic decrease in blood pressure.

SERENDIPITY, A SLOW ELEVATOR, AND SCIENTIFIC DISCOVERY

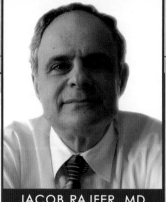

JACOB RAJFER, MD

In a strange twist of fate, a balky elevator led to the discovery of the link between nitric oxide (NO) and erections.

In late 1988, Dr. Jacob Rajfer, professor of urology at UCLA School of Medicine, had left a meeting on the school's second floor and was returning to his office on the sixth floor. **"I was trying to hitch a ride on the service elevator that takes the contaminated trash down into the basement,"** Dr. Rajfer recalls. **"It was a very slow elevator with doors that stay open too long— we'd been complaining about it for years."**

Dr. Rajfer stepped inside and pressed the button. As he waited, a sign on the lab directly across the corridor caught his attention. **"It read 'Vascular Smooth Muscle Lab' or something like that,"** recalls Dr. Rajfer. As the elevator door started closing, **"I put out my hand to stop it and walked back out. It was totally serendipitous."**

Dr. Rajfer had a special interest in vascular smooth muscle. Research had shown that an unidentified substance dubbed endothelium-derived relaxing factor, or EDRF, dilated blood vessels by relaxing smooth muscle. And it was known that erections resulted from vasodilation in the penis.

"Since the penis was full of vascular smooth muscle," says Dr. Rajfer, **"I figured penile erection worked very similarly to the way the blood vessels in the rest of the body work."** Indeed, he already had conducted studies showing that EDRF caused relaxation of rat penile smooth muscle cells that he had cultured in the laboratory.

When Dr. Rajfer stepped into the lab, he saw a technician hunched over a bench. He introduced himself, learned that the lab worked on vascular physiology, and asked whether they had heard of a compound called EDRF. They certainly had. **"The technician said, 'The guy who runs this lab recently wrote a paper stating that he thinks EDRF might be nitric oxide,'"** remembers Dr. Rajfer. The researcher was Dr. Louis Ignarro, a pharmacologist, who went on to win the Nobel Prize for the discovery of NO's role in smooth muscle relaxation (see page 21). Dr. Rajfer made an appointment to see him.

"When I opened his door at the appointed time, I said, 'Dr. Ignarro, my name is Jacob Rajfer, I'm a urologist here at UCLA, and I think I know why guys get erections.' He said, 'Please sit down.' We collaborated, and the rest is history."

In 1990, they published the first article showing that NO mediates erections, based on studies involving rabbits.[13] Then, in January 1992, their article in *The New England Journal of Medicine* appeared, showing that NO caused smooth-muscle relaxation in human corporal cavernosal tissue.[16] The chemical that leads to erections had been identified—thanks in part to a tired elevator door.

which in turn stimulates production of vessel-dilating cGMP.

Knowledge of NO's role in erections had important implications for the Pfizer scientists who would be designing the sildenafil clinical trials. Before sildenafil could enhance cGMP, NO had to trigger the biochemical erection process—and the release of NO depended on a signal from the nervous system that was usually cued by sexual stimulation.

"We realized," says Dr. Osterloh, "that our subjects had to be sexually stimulated for Viagra to be effective." So it was decided that men would be given either sildenafil or a placebo and then asked to view erotic videos or magazines; their erections were monitored with a device called the RigiScan. The RigiScan detects changes in penile

would record when they had erections, whether the erections resulted from sexual stimulation, and how firm the erections were. At the end of the week, the men would be admitted to a ward and then, following their last dose, they would view erotic material for 2 hours while being monitored with RigiScans.

A Prescription for Failure?

But despite the go-ahead for the study, expectations for success were quite low. After all, those "side effect" erections in earlier studies occurred with sildenafil doses of up to 100 mg taken 3 times a day. The dose chosen for this study—25 mg taken 3 times a day—was the maximum tolerated dose, but it had never been associated with erections. A higher dose might be needed to get a response.

The RigiScan, first marketed in 1985, was originally developed to monitor penile rigidity during uninterrupted sleep. Presence or absence of nocturnal erections can help determine whether ED is caused by psychological or physical factors.[17] In general, men with ED due to psychological causes are capable of erections while sleeping, and men with ED due to organic causes are not. For the first 2 pilot studies of sildenafil citrate as a treatment for ED, Dr. Mike Allen and Dr. Mitra Boolell of the early clinical research group at Pfizer, along with Dr. Clive Gingell of the University of Bristol, adapted the RigiScan to detect erections while men were conscious and viewing erotic materials.

tumescence and had been used to differentiate organic from psychogenic erectile dysfunction.[17] In addition, audiovisual sexual stimulation had been an accepted tool in psychological and therapeutic studies that required erotic stimuli. Dr. Mike Allen and other researchers at Pfizer-Sandwich merged these 2 approaches to assess the effects of sildenafil on ED very early in the development of Viagra.

The first study of sildenafil for treating ED would begin in Bristol, England, in late 1993. It was to be a double-blind, placebo-controlled, crossover trial in which 16 men with ED would take tablets 3 times a day for a week on an outpatient basis.[6] The men would also keep diaries in which they

But when the data were analyzed on completion of the study, it was obvious that sildenafil had made a difference. "Results from both the RigiScan and the diaries were very encouraging and showed a clear difference between the treatment and placebo," notes Dr. Osterloh. "There was also some feedback from patients saying, 'This was helpful, please send me some more tablets.'"

The positive results from this first ED study justified a second pilot study, also conducted in Bristol and again using RigiScans. This double-blind placebo-controlled study began in early 1994 and involved 12 men with ED who received a single dose of 10-, 25-, or 50-mg sildenafil or placebo.[18]

SILDENAFIL PILOT STUDY RESULTS[18]

The first pilot studies of sildenafil as a treatment for ED, carried out in Bristol, England, encouraged Pfizer to support the large-scale, pre–FDA approval clinical trials—eventually involving nearly 4500 men—that would make Viagra the world's first oral drug for the treatment of ED.

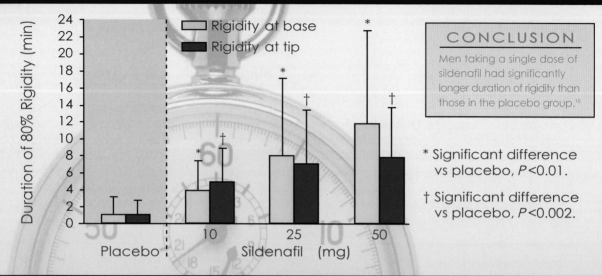

CONCLUSION

Men taking a single dose of sildenafil had significantly longer duration of rigidity than those in the placebo group.[18]

* Significant difference vs placebo, $P<0.01$.

† Significant difference vs placebo, $P<0.002$.

PERSPECTIVE FROM THE AUTHOR OF THE PILOT STUDIES: DR. MITRA BOOLELL, PFIZER CENTRAL RESEARCH–SANDWICH

It's quite difficult to change indications completely when you have a compound in development. In addition to a lot of persuading, it requires a scientific rationale and some convincing data—and we had very little of either in 1993.

We were fortunate in that at about the same time evidence was beginning to emerge in the literature that suggested a key role for nitric oxide in penile erection. Since these articles came at roughly the same time we were getting those anecdotal reports of erections, it provided a rationale for those observations.

But then, with only a small budget, we had to design a study that would convince people at Pfizer to investigate this new indication. Luckily, my manager, Dr. Mike Allen, and I had both graduated from the University of Bristol, so

we were able to collaborate with Dr. Clive Gingell, a urologist in Bristol whom we knew from our medical student days. Together we came up with the idea of testing sildenafil on patients using the RigiScan coupled with "blue" movies.

Since sildenafil works only when there is sexual stimulation, we needed a standardized technique for providing more or less the same degree of stimulation—and that basically meant getting patients to watch blue movies. In the UK, the laws that govern sexually explicit materials are very strict, and it was quite difficult for us to get permission to import this material from Europe.

Then we had to find a relaxed setting, the optimal environment for patients to respond. We couldn't run that kind of study in the average hospital environment. So we negotiated

to use a private hospital room and run the study in the evenings and on weekends to ensure privacy for the patients.

I phoned Dr. Sam Gepi-Attee, the research fellow, at the end of the first RigiScan study and asked him, "Do you think it's working?" He said, "Of course, it's working. These patients are phoning me that they want more tablets and saying this has changed their lives." In fact, the patients' partners were calling too. So there was a very strong message from the patients, even before we analyzed the results.

After that, the whole organization got very excited, and within just a few weeks of completing the RigiScan studies, we had put together an entire clinical research program for this new indication.

A PERSONAL PERSPECTIVE:
DR. PETER ELLIS

Q: You played a major role in the early research on Viagra. What has been the most rewarding result of the work you've done in making this drug available?

A: I've been very gratified by the letters we've received at Pfizer. I think I'm safe in saying we have hundreds of letters on file from patients expressing their gratitude for Viagra. Some of the most interesting letters were from the early days, when we were running our first clinical trials. The way a trial works is that patients will enroll for the length of the trial, and at the end of that time they must return all their unused tablets.

We had patients who, toward the end of the 3-month trial, were saying, **"Look, this is like throwing a drowning man a life preserver and then suddenly pulling the plug out of it. You have radically altered my life, things have never been so good for my family and me, and now you're taking it away. Please, can I continue on this drug?"**

We had many, many letters like that, where people were asking if they could stay on the drug. This was integral to our decision, early in the clinical program, to run what are called open-label extension trials.

Drug companies don't usually like doing them, because "open label" means no placebo control. So if a side effect is observed, you can't say, "Well, that wasn't the result of the drug, it would have happened anyway." But the patients were so vocal—they told us over and over, "We have to be allowed to stay on this drug now that you've given it to us." And the open-label extension trials did provide the opportunity to obtain long-term Viagra exposure data.

So by the time we filed for approval of Viagra, we had some patients who had been on the drug for up to 3 years. These were mainly the early patients, who started on this drug back in 1994 and did not wish to come off it again.

FROM TID TO PRN

"In all studies up until then, we were giving the drug 3 times a day. We knew as a practical matter that we couldn't administer it that often," recalls Dr. Peter Ellis, currently a senior project manager in the experimental medicine/early clinical group at Pfizer and one of the key leaders of the sildenafil research program.

But few at Pfizer believed that a single dose could be effective. Some scientists noted that erections had never been reported when sildenafil was taken just once a day. Even when the drug was given several times a day, spontaneous erections were noted only after the third or fourth day, suggesting the need for chronic dosing so that the drug could accumulate in tissues.

Once again, the skeptics were proven wrong. "By the time the second RigiScan study was completed in May 1994, we had data that showed that a single tablet—one single dose of Viagra—could promote erections in men who had ED," says Dr. Ellis. "This was when we positively thought, 'Okay, this could really be something worth having.'" ●

Louis J. Ignarro, PhD, receiving the Nobel Prize. Dr. Ignarro is 1 of 3 American scientists who won the 1998 Nobel Prize in Physiology or Medicine for the discovery of nitric oxide's role in human physiology. One of his contributions was to help elucidate the role of nitric oxide in erections, which is key to understanding how Viagra (sildenafil citrate) works.

FACTOID *To produce an erection, arterial blood flow into the penis increases enormously—from 1 mL/min to 25 mL/min.*

3

HOW VIAGRA WORKS

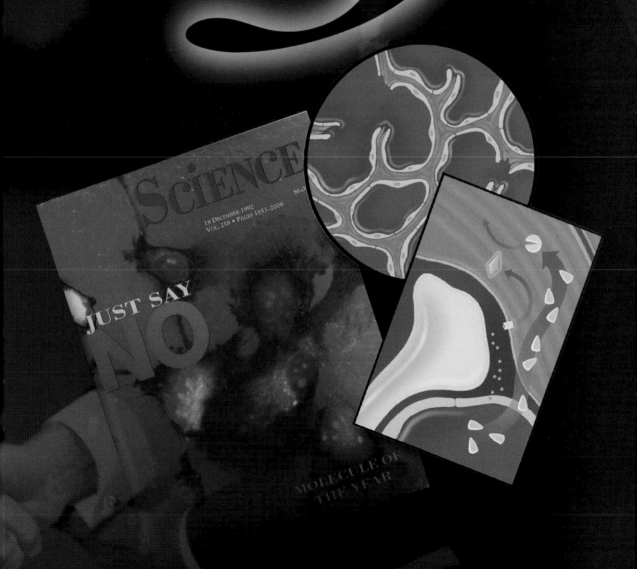

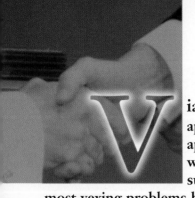

Viagra (sildenafil citrate) represented an entirely new approach to treating erectile dysfunction (ED). Before Viagra's approval by the FDA on March 27, 1998, treatment for ED was limited to injections into the penis, vacuum pumps, or surgery. With Viagra, men may obtain relief from one of their most vexing problems by swallowing a tablet that exerts its dramatic effect through an elegant biochemical strategem.

Today there is no mystery to Viagra. When pilot clinical studies began in 1993, Pfizer biologists' efforts to fully elucidate its mechanism of action were well under way. They already knew that Viagra inhibited phosphodiesterase type 5 (PDE 5). After first reports of erections in 1992, Pfizer scientists began looking for evidence of PDE 5 in the penis. In 1994, they successfully isolated PDE 5 from human corpus cavernosal tissue, helping to confirm their belief that sildenafil caused erections by inhibiting PDE 5 in penile tissue.[12,19] Knowing that sildenafil blocked PDE 5—

and that PDE 5 was present in the penis—Pfizer scientists suspected that the drug must aid erections by helping cyclic guanosine monophosphate (cGMP) accumulate. Viagra was found to be extremely specific in its action: It selectively and strongly inhibits PDE 5, which is found in highest concentrations in the penis.[12,20]

ANATOMY OF AN ERECTION

Certainly from a man's perspective, the transformation of his penis from flaccid to erect is a

PENILE ANATOMY: BLOOD VESSELS AND EXPANDABLE SPACES

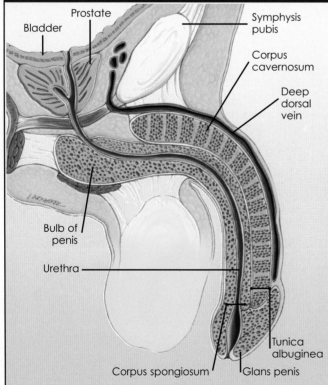

Bladder
Prostate
Symphysis pubis
Corpus cavernosum
Deep dorsal vein
Bulb of penis
Urethra
Tunica albuginea
Corpus spongiosum
Glans penis

The penis consists almost entirely of 2 erectile chambers, collectively called the corpora cavernosa, which in turn are filled with hollow spaces called sinusoids. The penile artery supplies the corpora cavernosa through small vessels known as the helicine arteries or arterioles. The tunica albuginea is a dense, fibrous elastic covering for the corpora cavernosa. In the flaccid state, smooth muscle cells in the corpora cavernosa are contracted, keeping arteries and sinusoids small. During an erection, the smooth muscle cells relax and blood flow is increased tremendously into the corpora cavernosa, causing the sinusoids to fill with blood and swell. The tunica albuginea compresses small penile veins, thereby trapping blood in the penis so it remains erect.

NITRIC OXIDE:
A DISCOVERY WORTHY OF A NOBEL PRIZE

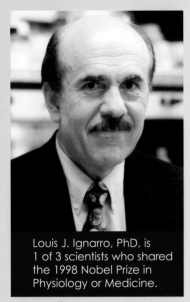

Louis J. Ignarro, PhD, is 1 of 3 scientists who shared the 1998 Nobel Prize in Physiology or Medicine.

Nitric oxide's crucial role—in causing erections and in human physiology in general—has been appreciated for only about a dozen years.

Nitric oxide (NO) was once regarded mainly as an undesirable air pollutant responsible for forming ozone. But researchers in recent years have found that molecules of NO are responsible for a wide variety of critical bodily functions, including nerve transmission, immunity, and—crucial for erections—smooth muscle relaxation.

The discovery of NO's role in making smooth muscles relax was considered so significant that the 3 scientists responsible were awarded the 1998 Nobel Prize in Physiology or Medicine. Winners included Dr. Louis J. Ignarro (pictured), distinguished professor of pharmacology at the University of California at Los Angeles. The other Nobel winners were Dr. Robert F. Furchgott and Dr. Ferid Murad.

In addition, the journal *Science* named NO "molecule of the year" in 1992.

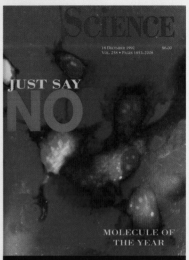

By 1992, the newly discovered knowledge about NO's role in human physiology made this molecule—NO—the cover story for the journal *Science*.

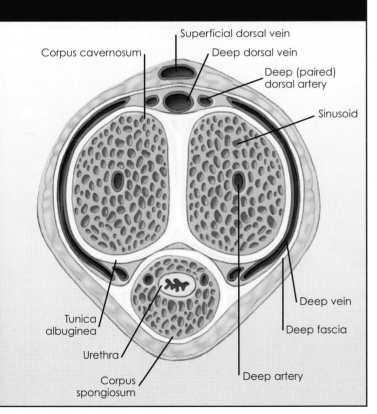

- Corpus cavernosum
- Superficial dorsal vein
- Deep dorsal vein
- Deep (paired) dorsal artery
- Sinusoid
- Deep vein
- Deep fascia
- Deep artery
- Corpus spongiosum
- Urethra
- Tunica albuginea

remarkable metamorphosis. But from a physiologic standpoint, the way in which a penis becomes erect during sexual activity represents a triumphant mixture of nerves, arteries, muscle fibers, blood, hormones, and other chemicals, and a dash of erotic stimuli.

The penis consists almost entirely of 2 parallel erection chambers, which are known collectively as the corpora cavernosa. This spongy erectile tissue is made up of a network of tiny arteries and hollow spaces, or sinusoids. Most of the time, only a trickle of blood flows within the penis, since these arteries and sinusoids are tightly constricted by muscles: the smooth muscles making up the walls of the penile arteries and a network of smooth muscles forming the boundaries of the sinusoids.

THE ERECTILE CYCLE:

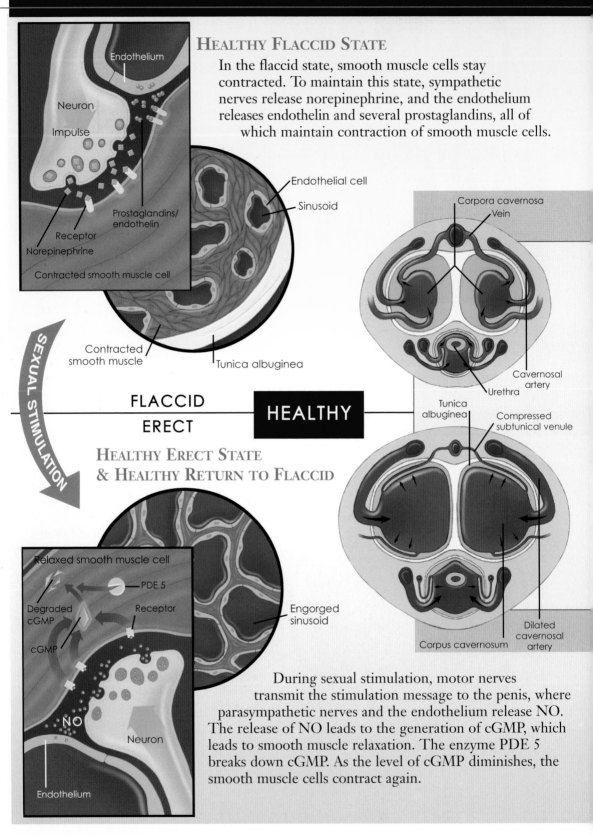

HEALTHY FLACCID STATE

In the flaccid state, smooth muscle cells stay contracted. To maintain this state, sympathetic nerves release norepinephrine, and the endothelium releases endothelin and several prostaglandins, all of which maintain contraction of smooth muscle cells.

Endothelium

Neuron

Impulse

Prostaglandins/
endothelin

Receptor

Norepinephrine

Contracted smooth muscle cell

Endothelial cell

Sinusoid

Contracted
smooth muscle

Tunica albuginea

Corpora cavernosa
Vein

Cavernosal
artery

Urethra

FLACCID

ERECT

HEALTHY

SEXUAL STIMULATION

HEALTHY ERECT STATE
& HEALTHY RETURN TO FLACCID

Relaxed smooth muscle cell

PDE 5

Degraded
cGMP

Receptor

cGMP

NO

Neuron

Endothelium

Engorged
sinusoid

Tunica
albuginea

Compressed
subtunical venule

Dilated
cavernosal
artery

Corpus cavernosum

During sexual stimulation, motor nerves transmit the stimulation message to the penis, where parasympathetic nerves and the endothelium release NO. The release of NO leads to the generation of cGMP, which leads to smooth muscle relaxation. The enzyme PDE 5 breaks down cGMP. As the level of cGMP diminishes, the smooth muscle cells contract again.

ERECTILE DYSFUNCTION

In men with erectile dysfunction, not enough NO may be produced to overcome PDE 5 and allow the accumulation of cGMP. Smooth muscle cells stay contracted despite sexual stimulation.

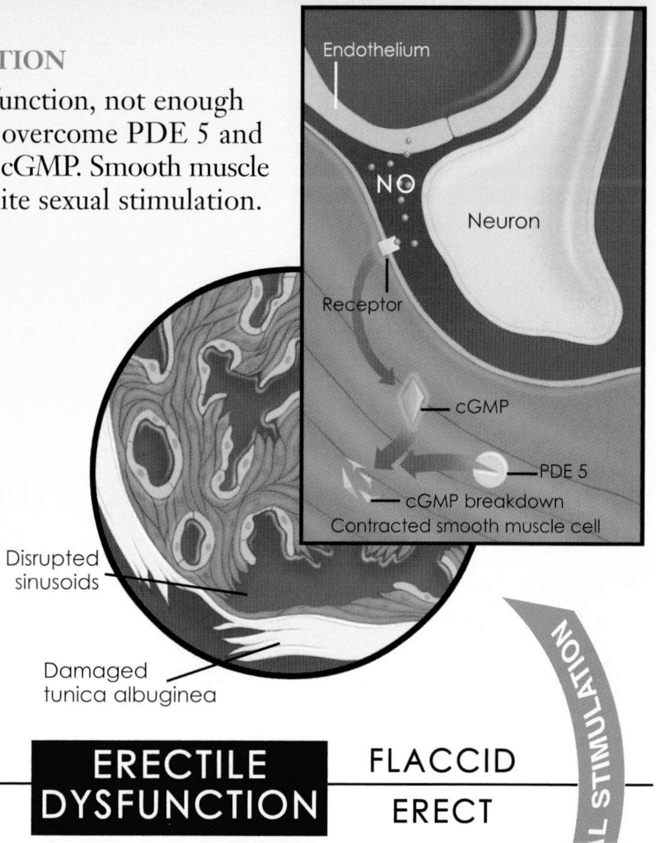

Endothelium

NO

Neuron

Receptor

cGMP

PDE 5

cGMP breakdown

Contracted smooth muscle cell

Disrupted sinusoids

Damaged tunica albuginea

HYDRAULICS OF ERECTION

The smooth muscle lining penile arteries normally keeps those arteries constricted, severely limiting blood flow into the penis. An erection occurs when sexual excitement produces chemicals that signal smooth muscles to relax, causing penile arteries to dilate and allowing blood to rush in and fill the corpora cavernosa. At the same time, the penile veins are compressed by the tunica albuginea to prevent the outflow of blood.

ERECTILE DYSFUNCTION

FLACCID

ERECT

SEXUAL STIMULATION

ERECTION AFTER TREATMENT WITH VIAGRA

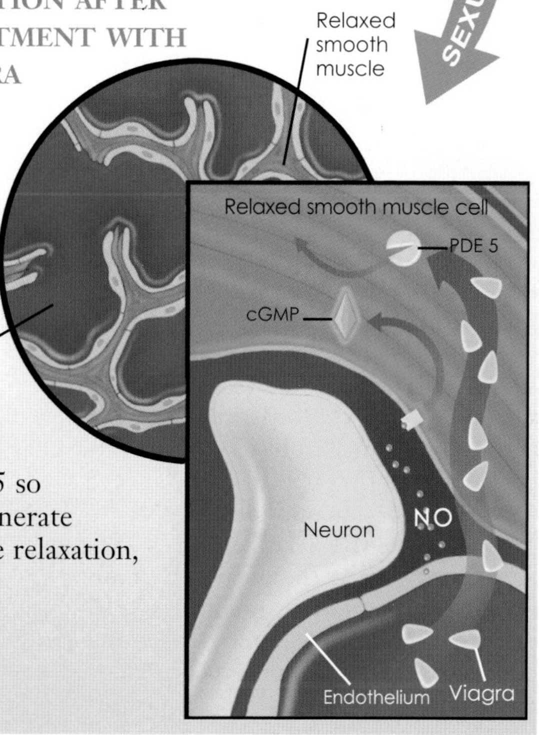

Relaxed smooth muscle

Relaxed smooth muscle cell

PDE 5

cGMP

Engorged and disrupted sinusoids

Neuron

NO

Endothelium   Viagra

Viagra inhibits the production of PDE 5 so that even small amounts of NO can generate enough cGMP to allow smooth muscle relaxation, making an erection possible.

For an erection to occur, the trickle of blood in the penis must turn into a torrent. That can only happen if those intrapenile smooth muscles ease their grip, allowing the penile arteries to dilate and the sinusoids to expand. Next a surge of blood can enter, transforming the flaccid penis into an erection.

Producing a successful (non-nocturnal) erection requires erotic stimuli, which can range from the indirect (a whiff of perfume) to the highly direct (stroking of the penis itself); a nervous system capable of translating those erotic stimuli into nerve impulses and transmitting them to the penis; and the right balance of hormones and healthy arteries capable of both dilating and retaining their infusion of erectile blood. But perhaps the most crucial of all requirements for a successful erection are the chemicals that widen the penile arteries so the blood responsible for erections can flow in.

NITRIC OXIDE'S CRUCIAL ROLE

Nitric oxide (NO) is the chemical that literally launches a man's erection, since it causes his penile arteries to dilate.[13]

The dilation necessary for erections is the culmination of a sequence of events beginning with the excitement phase of male sexual response: Erotic stimuli are transformed into nerve impulses that race down the spinal cord to the penis itself. When these impulses reach the nerve endings in the penis, NO is released.

NO acts as a neurotransmitter, delivering the message of sexual arousal throughout the smooth muscle cells lining the penile artery walls and those surrounding the penile sinusoids. The smooth muscle cells respond by relaxing, but NO does not cause muscle relaxation by itself. Instead, NO molecules combine with the enzyme guanylate cyclase to instruct each smooth muscle cell to begin producing cGMP, a key chemical messenger in the body.[20,21] As the muscle cells along the penile arteries start to produce cGMP, these previously constricted arteries start to expand, allowing the inrushing of blood that causes an erection.

CYCLIC GMP BUILDS UP AND IS BROKEN DOWN

As long as cGMP levels are maintained, blood will keep flowing to the penis and the erection will be maintained. Ejaculation or the cessation of sexual stimulation ends an erection by signaling cGMP production to grind to an abrupt halt.

But even before ejaculation, cGMP levels—and thus a man's erection—may be jeopardized by the enzyme PDE 5, which the penis produces to prevent itself from staying permanently erect. PDE 5 breaks down the erection-building cGMP molecules.[20] Getting and maintaining an erection requires the proper balance between cGMP's production and its degradation by PDE 5.

PDE 5 AND ERECTILE DYSFUNCTION

PDE 5, by degrading cGMP, contributes to erectile dysfunction in millions of men. These are men whose cGMP levels—for a variety of reasons that probably include impaired NO production—are reduced. Because PDE 5 diminishes their already low levels of cGMP, these men cannot obtain a level of cGMP high enough to initiate or maintain an erection.

For the millions of men afflicted with ED who thought there was no hope for their condition, this is where Viagra can intervene. By inhibiting PDE 5, Viagra allows erection-producing cGMP molecules to accumulate to levels high enough to create and maintain an erection.

WHY VIAGRA ACTS SO SPECIFICALLY

PDE 5, the body's key erection-limiting chemical, differs from all other phosphodiesterases in a crucial respect: **PDE 5 is found in highest concentrations in penile tissue.[20] Thus the fact that Viagra specifically blocks PDE 5 explains how it can be so potent as a treatment for ED.**

Viagra's mechanism of action is unique, and its method of administration, a pill, is convenient and allows men with ED to respond to sexual stimulation. ●

RELATIVE SPECIFICITY OF VIAGRA (SILDENAFIL CITRATE) TO INHIBIT PDE ISOZYMES

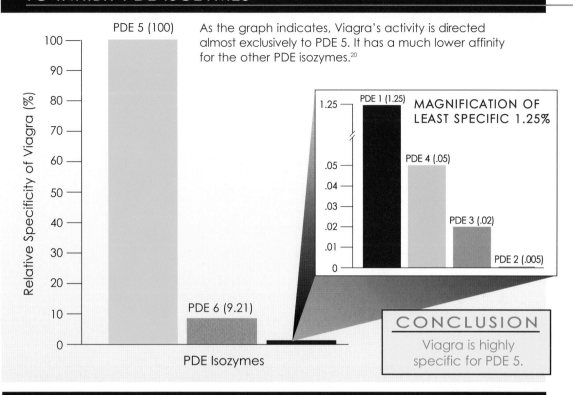

As the graph indicates, Viagra's activity is directed almost exclusively to PDE 5. It has a much lower affinity for the other PDE isozymes.[20]

MAGNIFICATION OF LEAST SPECIFIC 1.25%

PDE 1 (1.25)
PDE 4 (.05)
PDE 3 (.02)
PDE 2 (.005)

PDE 5 (100)
PDE 6 (9.21)

Relative Specificity of Viagra (%)

PDE Isozymes

CONCLUSION
Viagra is highly specific for PDE 5.

WELL-CHARACTERIZED PHOSPHODIESTERASES[20*]

FAMILY	TISSUE LOCALIZATION
PDE 1	Brain, heart, kidney, liver, skeletal muscle, vascular and visceral smooth muscle
PDE 2	Adrenal cortex, brain, corpus cavernosum, heart, kidney, liver, visceral smooth muscle, skeletal muscle
PDE 3	Corpus cavernosum, heart, platelets, vascular and visceral smooth muscle, liver, kidney
PDE 4	Kidney, lung, mast cells, heart, skeletal muscle, vascular and visceral smooth muscle
PDE 5	Corpus cavernosum, platelets, skeletal muscle, vascular and visceral smooth muscle
PDE 6	Retina

*PDEs 7–11 have been identified but are still being characterized as of 2000.

Viagra (sildenafil citrate) had shown that it could produce erections in small numbers of men with erectile dysfunction while they watched erotic videos and were hooked up to RigiScans. But how could it be tested in thousands of men right in the *bedroom,* where men and their partners would actually use it? The answer proved to be patient diaries and efficacy assessment instruments.

Pfizer SIL
Vis

INVESTIGATOR

PLEASE USE

INVESTIGATOR

DATE OF VISIT 9 /18 / 96
(month/day/year)

PLEASE USE A CROSS MARK ⊠ WHERE APPLICABLE AND BE SURE TO INITIAL AND DATE ALL CORRECTIONS

Journal des activités sexuelles

Pfizer SILDENAFIL
Visit: WEEK 4

SUBJECT INITIALS

PROTOCOL #	INVESTIGATOR	
1 0 6	2 5 5 8	SUBJECT I.D./ RANDOMIZATION #
1 4 8	9 0 0 3	
DRUG CODE	SUBJECT ENTRY #	

INVESTIGATOR

DATE OF VISIT OCT / 26/ 96
(month/day/year)

PLEASE USE A CROSS MARK ⊠ WHERE APPLICABLE AND BE SURE TO INITIAL AND DATE ALL CORRECTIONS

Journal des activités sexuelles

Veuiller répondre aux questions suivantes le plus honnêtement et le plus clairement possible à chaque fois que vous prenez une dose du médicament à l'étude ou que vous avez des rapports sexuels. Utilisez les définitions suivantes pour répondre aux questions :

- **stimulation sexuelle :** comprend toutes les situations telles que les jeux amoureux (caresses, stimulations érotiques) avec une partenaire, qui généralement entrainent une excitation sexuelle et une érection.

- **rapport sexuel réussi** se définit comme une activité sexuelle comportant une pénétration vaginale (introduction du pénis dans le vagin) et que vous penser être satisfaisante (e.g. votre érection est suffisamment rigide et dure suffisamment longtemps).

Date (mois/jour/année)	9 / 15 / 96
	COCHEZ UNE BOÎTE
1a. Est-ce que la médication a l'étude a été prise ?	(1) ☒ Oui (2) ☐ Non
1b. Si oui, s'il vous plaît indiquer le nombre de comprimés pris.	I
	COCHEZ UNE BOÎTE
2. Avez-vous eu une stimulation sexuelle?	(1) ☒ Oui (2) ☐ Non
	COCHEZ UNE BOÎTE
3. Avez-vous eu un rapport sexuel réussi?	(1) ☐ Oui (2) ☒ Non

Appendix 14.2.1

**Erectile D
(EDITS)
Partner V**
(Final Novembe

Subject ID Nu

Today's Date:

What   treat

FACTOID *The average frequency of Viagra use by men in the clinical trials was twice per week.*

i) Very satisfied
ii) Satisfied
iii) Neither satisfied nor dissatisfied
iv) Dissatisfied
v) Very dissatisfied

2. During the past four weeks, to what degree has the treatment met your expectations?
i) Completely
ii) Considerably
iii) Half way
iv) A little
v) Not at all

VIAGRA CLINICAL RESEARCH: THE BEHIND-THE-SCENES STORY

4

FIL
Week 2

SUBJECT INITIALS

PROTOCOL #
1 0 3
0 1 4 8
DRUG CODE

INVESTIGATOR
9 5 0 0
9 0
SUBJECT ENTRY #

SUBJECT
RANDOMIZATION #

MAY, 5, 99
CHECK ONE BOX

DATE OF VISIT
(month/day/year)
7 10 96

...ion taken?
⊘ Yes
☐ No

...the number

...MARK ☒ WHERE APPLICABLE AND BE SURE TO <u>INITIAL</u> AND <u>DATE</u> ALL CORRECTIONS

CHECK ONE BOX
...al stimulation:
☐ Yes
☐ No

...lowing questions as honestly and clearly as possible every time you take the study
...ve sexual intercourse. In answering these questions, the following definitions apply

...on includes any situations, including foreplay and caressing, that you would expect to lead
...al and an erection.

...al intercourse is sexual activity which involves vaginal penetration and which you found
..., your erection is hard enough and lasts long enough).

CHECK ONE BOX
...ul sexual intercourse?
☐ Yes
☐ No, erection was not hard
did not last long enough
☐ No, other reasons

...ay/year):
_____ / _

CHEC
...study medication taken?
☑ Yes
☐ No

...ease indicate the number
...taken:
_____

CHEC
...ave any sexual stimulation:
☑ Yes
☐ No

CHEC
...ave successful sexual intercourse?
☑ Yes
☐ No, erectio...
did not last...
☐ No, other...

...ction Inventory of Treatment Sa...

...n

_____

_____

method   is   your   husband/partner

_____

INTERNATIONAL INDEX OF ERECTILE FUNCTION (IIE

OVER THE PAST 4 WEEKS .

1. How often were you able to get an erection during sexual activity?
   0 = No sexual activity   1 = Almost never/never   2 = A few times (much less than h
   3 = Sometimes (about half the time)   4 = Most times (much more than half the time

2. When you had erections with sexual stimulation, how often were your er
   for penetration?
   0 = No sexual activity   1 = Almost never/never   2 = A few times (much less than h
   3 = Sometimes (about half the time)   4 = Most times (much more than half the time

3. When you attempted sexual intercourse, how often were you able to per
   0 = Did not attempt intercourse   1 = Almost never/never   2 = A few times (much le
   3 = Sometimes (about half the time)   4 = Most times (much more than half the time

4. During sexual intercourse, how often were you able to maintain your er
   penetrated (entered) your partner?
   0 = Did not attempt intercourse   1 = Almost never/never   2 = A few times (much le
   3 = Sometimes (about half the time)   4 = Most times (much more than half the time

5. During sexual intercourse, how difficult was it to maintain your erection t
   0 = Did not attempt intercourse   1 = Extremely difficult   2 = Very difficult   3 = Diffi
   4 = Slightly difficult   5 = Not difficult

6. How many times have you attempted sexual intercourse?
   0 = No attempts   1 = One to two attempts   2 = Three to four attempts
   3 = Five to six attempts   4 = Seven to ten attempts   5 = Eleven-plus attempts

7. When you attempted sexual intercourse, how often was it satisfactory fo
   0 = Did not attempt intercourse   1 = Almost never/never   2 = A few times (much le
   3 = Sometimes (about half the time)   4 = Most times (much more than half the time

8. How much have you enjoyed sexual intercourse?
   0 = No intercourse   1 = No enjoyment   2 = Not very enjoyable   3 = Fairly enjoyab
   4 = Highly enjoyable   5 = Very highly enjoyable

9. When you had sexual stimulation or intercourse, how often did you ejacu
   0 = No sexual stimulation/intercourse   1 = Almost never/never   2 = A few times (mu
   3 = Sometimes (about half the time)   4 = Most times (much more than half the time)

10. When you had sexual stimulation or intercourse, how often did you have the
    0 = No sexual stimulation/intercourse   1 = Almost never/never   2 = A few times (mu
    3 = Sometimes (about half the time)   4 = Most times (much more than half the time)

11. How often have you felt sexual desire?

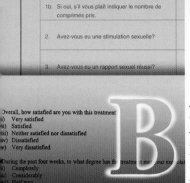

y May 1994, results of the pilot studies were in. A single dose of Viagra (sildenafil citrate) seemed capable of producing erections in men with erectile dysfunction (ED). But even then, the fate of what would come to be known as the world's first oral medication for ED was by no means assured.

The first key challenge was a matter of methodology: how to prove that an oral drug can alleviate ED. This had never been done before. The RigiScan had provided useful data about Viagra in a laboratory setting, but now the doctors at Pfizer had to determine whether the medication worked under real-life conditions: in the bedroom, where changes in erectile function could not be monitored with objective devices like the RigiScan. Pfizer scientists realized they needed an instrument that could accurately reflect improvements in erectile ability. After consulting with several experts, they concluded that the right instrument would be a questionnaire, but the right questionnaire did not exist.

A lucky break occurred in 1994, when Dr. Osterloh attended the annual meeting of the American Urological Association. He went to a poster session where a urologist reported on a sexual-function questionnaire that he was developing but that had not yet been validated.

CREATING AN INSTRUMENT TO MEASURE ED

With input from his colleagues in Sandwich and academic experts, Dr. Osterloh built upon these questions to create the International Index of Erectile Function (IIEF), a 15-item questionnaire that now serves as the standard measure for assessing the effectiveness of ED treatments. But validating the IIEF—showing that the questions were universally understood and that the responses accurately reflected the clinical findings—would prove to be a major challenge requiring international collaboration.

At the beginning of the validation effort, ED patients and their partners in 5 countries were interviewed to discover the domains of "male sexual function" that people in different cultures could agree upon. The interviewers found 4 domains that seemed universally accepted: erectile function, orgasmic function, sexual desire, and intercourse satisfaction.[22] (Another domain, overall satisfaction, was added later.)

The IIEF was pilot-tested on men with ED in the United Kingdom and Sweden and then was linguistically validated in 12 countries in 10 languages. Finally, it was proven scientifically and clinically sound in clinical studies using the very specific and accepted methods for determining the validity of a scientific questionnaire. For example, one study demonstrated that the IIEF was able

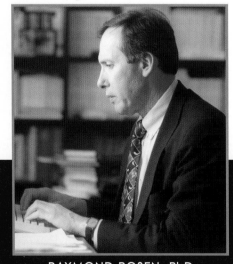

One of those instrumental in validating the IIEF was Dr. Raymond Rosen, professor of psychiatry at the University of Medicine and Dentistry of New Jersey–Robert Wood Johnson Medical School in Piscataway, New Jersey. "Previous self-assessments of sexual functioning were too long and complex for patients and had not been validated psychometrically, culturally, or linguistically," says Dr. Rosen.

RAYMOND ROSEN, PhD

INTERNATIONAL INDEX OF ERECTILE FUNCTION (IIEF) QUESTIONNAIRE

OVER THE PAST 4 WEEKS . . .

1. How often were you able to get an erection during sexual activity?
   0 = No sexual activity   1 = Almost never/never   2 = A few times (much less than half the time)
   3 = Sometimes (about half the time)   4 = Most times (much more than half the time)   5 = Almost always/always

2. When you had erections with sexual stimulation, how often were your erections hard enough for penetration?
   0 = No sexual activity   1 = Almost never/never   2 = A few times (much less than half the time)
   3 = Sometimes (about half the time)   4 = Most times (much more than half the time)   5 = Almost always/always

3. When you attempted sexual intercourse, how often were you able to penetrate (enter) your partner?
   0 = Did not attempt intercourse   1 = Almost never/never   2 = A few times (much less than half the time)
   3 = Sometimes (about half the time)   4 = Most times (much more than half the time)   5 = Almost always/always

4. During sexual intercourse, how often were you able to maintain your erection after you had penetrated (entered) your partner?
   0 = Did not attempt intercourse   1 = Almost never/never   2 = A few times (much less than half the time)
   3 = Sometimes (about half the time)   4 = Most times (much more than half the time)   5 = Almost always/always

5. During sexual intercourse, how difficult was it to maintain your erection to completion of intercourse?
   0 = Did not attempt intercourse   1 = Extremely difficult   2 = Very difficult   3 = Difficult
   4 = Slightly difficult   5 = Not difficult

6. How many times have you attempted sexual intercourse?
   0 = No attempts   1 = One to two attempts   2 = Three to four attempts
   3 = Five to six attempts   4 = Seven to ten attempts   5 = Eleven-plus attempts

7. When you attempted sexual intercourse, how often was it satisfactory for you?
   0 = Did not attempt intercourse   1 = Almost never/never   2 = A few times (much less than half the time)
   3 = Sometimes (about half the time)   4 = Most times (much more than half the time)   5 = Almost always/always

8. How much have you enjoyed sexual intercourse?
   0 = No intercourse   1 = No enjoyment   2 = Not very enjoyable   3 = Fairly enjoyable
   4 = Highly enjoyable   5 = Very highly enjoyable

9. When you had sexual stimulation or intercourse, how often did you ejaculate?
   0 = No sexual stimulation/intercourse   1 = Almost never/never   2 = A few times (much less than half the time)
   3 = Sometimes (about half the time)   4 = Most times (much more than half the time)   5 = Almost always/always

10. When you had sexual stimulation or intercourse, how often did you have the feeling of orgasm or climax?
    0 = No sexual stimulation/intercourse   1 = Almost never/never   2 = A few times (much less than half the time)
    3 = Sometimes (about half the time)   4 = Most times (much more than half the time)   5 = Almost always/always

11. How often have you felt sexual desire?
    1 = Almost never/never   2 = A few times (much less than half the time)   3 = Sometimes (about half the time)
    4 = Most times (much more than half the time)   5 = Almost always/always

12. How would you rate your level of sexual desire?
    1 = Very low/none at all   2 = Low   3 = Moderate   4 = High   5 = Very high

13. How satisfied have you been with your overall sex life?
    1 = Very dissatisfied   2 = Moderately dissatisfied   3 = About equally satisfied
    and dissatisfied   4 = Moderately satisfied   5 = Very satisfied

14. How satisfied have you been with your sexual relationship with your partner?
    1 = Very dissatisfied   2 = Moderately dissatisfied   3 = About equally satisfied
    and dissatisfied   4 = Moderately satisfied   5 = Very satisfied

15. How do you rate your confidence that you could get and keep an erection?
    1 = Very low   2 = Low   3 = Moderate   4 = High   5 = Very high

DOMAINS OF SEXUAL FUNCTION
ERECTILE FUNCTION
INTERCOURSE SATISFACTION
ORGASMIC FUNCTION
SEXUAL DESIRE
OVERALL SATISFACTION

Between the time a drug is initially synthesized and the time it is finally approved for marketing, it generally goes through 3 types, or phases, of clinical trials. Once a drug is marketed, a fourth phase may be conducted as well. The 4 phases can be described as follows.

Phase 1: Carried out on a small number of healthy volunteers who do not have the health problem that the drug is designed to address. Volunteers are kept in a highly monitored environment, usually a hospital or clinic. *The main goals of a phase 1 trial are to assess safety for further human studies and to investigate the drug's pharmacokinetic profile and hemodynamic effects.*

Phase 2: Studies involving a small number of patients affected by the medical condition that the drug is intended to treat. As with phase 1 trials, these patients are usually tested in a closely monitored setting, such as a clinic. *Phase 2 trials are usually randomized, placebo-controlled, double-blind studies. The main goal is to help determine the dose that is both safe and effective in the patient population affected by the target condition.*

Phase 3: Large-scale randomized, placebo-controlled, double-blind studies involving usually hundreds of patients who have the health condition targeted for treatment. These patients take the drug in the setting in which it is intended to be used once marketed. *Phase 3 studies provide a wealth of data on a drug's safety and efficacy and are carried out using the dosages that the pharmaceutical company expects to include when it files its New Drug Application (NDA) with the FDA.* These efficacy and safety results form the basis for the final drug label. Companies may also initiate similar studies, called phase 3B trials, after they have submitted the NDA but before the drug is approved.

Phase 4: Clinical studies carried out after the drug is approved and marketed. *Phase 4 studies can help define how well the drug works in special situations or when used by specific patient populations.*

CLINICAL TRIALS IN THE PATIENT POPULATION AFFECTED BY THE TARGET CONDITION

to discriminate between men who had ED and those who did not.[22] In another study that enrolled ED patients, this instrument could accurately measure treatment-induced changes in these patients.[22]

HOW WOULD IT WORK IN THE FIELD?

Elated by the success of the 2 RigiScan studies, and reassured by other studies that had established the dose regimens that men could safely tolerate, Pfizer researchers were ready to shift sildenafil testing into high gear. While the 2 RigiScan studies had involved a total of only 28 men with ED, clinical testing would now move to large-scale phase 2 studies involving hundreds of ED patients.

The first large phase 2 study began in September 1994 and involved 351 ED patients enrolled at 37 centers in the United Kingdom, Sweden, and France. In this double-blind, placebo-controlled study, the men took 1 tablet daily of either a placebo or a 10-, 25-, or 50-mg dose of sildenafil for 4 weeks at home.[6,23]

"This study was designed primarily to ask, 'Does the drug work in outpatients?'" says Dr. Osterloh. "It had worked very well when men were lying still and watching films, but would it work in the normal situation at home? And we had other concerns as well, such as whether the placebo response would be high and whether there would be a dose-response relationship."

Results exceeded the most optimistic expectations. "The interim analysis that came out in February 1995 showed a beautiful dose response on the IIEF questions in general and on the key question of whether sildenafil improved men's erections," says Dr. Osterloh. "And the safety data also looked very good as well."

The second large-scale phase 2 trial, involving 233 ED patients in the United Kingdom, Norway, and

FREQUENCY OF ERECTIONS LASTING LONG ENOUGH FOR SEXUAL ACTIVITY

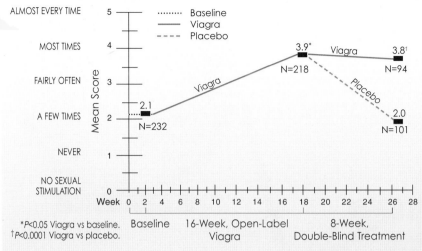

.... Baseline
——— Viagra
– – – Placebo

*P<0.05 Viagra vs baseline.
†P<0.0001 Viagra vs placebo.

Baseline | 16-Week, Open-Label Viagra | 8-Week, Double-Blind Treatment

After taking Viagra for 16 weeks, half of the men were blindly switched to placebo while the remainder continued on Viagra for another 8 weeks. The Pfizer team wanted to determine if Viagra's effects continued after patients stopped taking it.[6]

CONCLUSION

Men who stopped taking Viagra (the placebo group) saw their erectile function return to the level reported before the first dose.[6]

France,[24] began in December 1994, just 2 months after the first phase 2 trial.

"STEPPING UP" TO THE RIGHT DOSE

In contrast to the first large-scale trial, which involved a fixed dose and was double-blind, this was an open-label dose-escalation study. Men with ED were started on a 10-mg daily dose of sildenafil and periodically were allowed to stepwise increase their daily intake (to 25-, 50-, or 100-mg doses) if they were not helped by the lower dose and could tolerate the higher one.[24] Following 16 weeks of treatment came a "blind extension" phase in which those men responding to sildenafil were randomized to continue taking either their most recent dose of sildenafil or a matched placebo tablet.[6]

The good news: Sildenafil was proving to be extremely well tolerated, with most men in

SHEDDING LIGHT ON "PSYCHOGENIC" ED

As is customary in new drug development, the participants chosen for these early clinical studies were carefully selected for having the best chance for a successful outcome. The doctors at Pfizer assumed that organic ED would be more difficult to treat than psychogenic ED.

Therefore, outpatients enrolled in these first 2 large-scale phase 2 studies were primarily men whose ED had no detectable organic cause and presumably was psychogenic in nature. Others had ED of mixed causes—that is, psychological factors plus controlled hypertension or high cholesterol levels. The double-blind phase (see graph above) added to the second study would provide useful information about these men.

"Since most of these men had ED stemming from psychological causes, we thought that perhaps, after sildenafil gave them their confidence back, they wouldn't need further treatment and sildenafil would in effect result in a cure," says Dr. Osterloh. "So this study was designed to answer the question, Can you stop treating once you have treated successfully?" The answer to that latter question, says Dr. Osterloh, was a "quite surprising" but resounding "no."

"One investigator rang us up quite excited because he had deliberately not told the patient that he might be switched to a placebo, and the patient had called him to complain, 'The tablet has stopped working!'" says Dr. Osterloh. "Another patient reported that his wife got so angry when the tablets stopped working that she threw them into the fireplace."

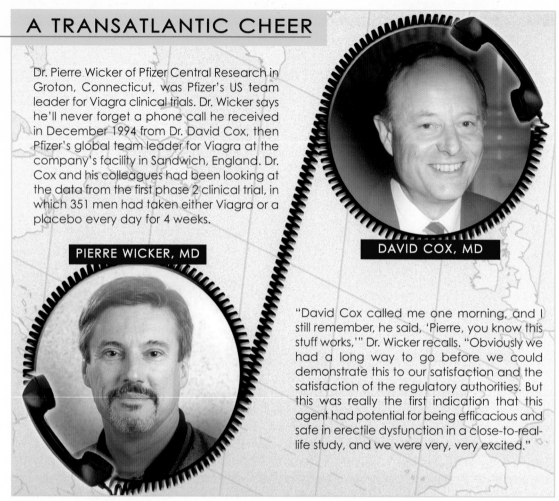

A TRANSATLANTIC CHEER

Dr. Pierre Wicker of Pfizer Central Research in Groton, Connecticut, was Pfizer's US team leader for Viagra clinical trials. Dr. Wicker says he'll never forget a phone call he received in December 1994 from Dr. David Cox, then Pfizer's global team leader for Viagra at the company's facility in Sandwich, England. Dr. Cox and his colleagues had been looking at the data from the first phase 2 clinical trial, in which 351 men had taken either Viagra or a placebo every day for 4 weeks.

PIERRE WICKER, MD

DAVID COX, MD

"David Cox called me one morning, and I still remember, he said, 'Pierre, you know this stuff works,'" Dr. Wicker recalls. "Obviously we had a long way to go before we could demonstrate this to our satisfaction and the satisfaction of the regulatory authorities. But this was really the first indication that this agent had potential for being efficacious and safe in erectile dysfunction in a close-to-real-life study, and we were very, very excited."

the dose-escalation trial opting for the top (100-mg) dose as their PRN dose. Some men did report adverse effects, primarily headache, flushing, and dyspepsia.[24]

This study also showed that the effect of sildenafil on ED generally could be detected soon after initiating treatment. And in the crossover to placebo part of the study, the same men who responded readily to sildenafil experienced rapid return to baseline erectile function.

Results of this open dose-escalation trial not only gave further evidence of safety and effectiveness but provided that information quickly. Notes Dr. Osterloh: "This was a very useful trial in the early-stage development of sildenafil because we got the data on how the drug was doing far earlier than with a double-blind trial, where you wait months for the results."

PHASE 2 STUDY RESULTS EXCEED EXPECTATIONS

"The results from these 2 studies were so positive—we had an 89% response rate with the 50-mg dose, for example—that we decided that all other trials would be expanded to include people whose ED was due to predominantly organic causes," says Dr. Osterloh. "We reasoned that even if the drug didn't work for them, it would have enough horsepower among people with psychogenically induced ED that we'd still be able to separate it from the placebo."

Additional phase 2 studies would also be carried out. Studies in Australia and Canada involved ED patients who were randomized to receive 50 mg, 100 mg, and—for the first time—200 mg of sildenafil. Results led Pfizer to abandon the 200-mg dose, since it proved no more effective than

THE PARTNER TEST

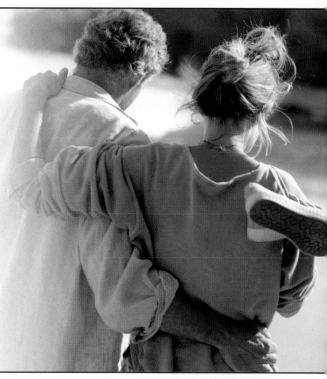

Another especially noteworthy aspect of the Viagra research involved the sexual partners of the men in the trials. **"We administered an abbreviated version of the IIEF to the partners starting with the very first trials,"** says Dr. Osterloh.

The 2 basic questions were "How do you rate your partner's erections" over the course of the study and "When you had sexual intercourse, how often was it satisfactory for you?" The answers provided valuable information to Pfizer's doctors: **"The partners corroborated the very positive assessments we were getting from patients who were treated with Viagra,"** says Dr. Osterloh.

100 mg and resulted in a greater frequency of side effects.[6] To obtain safety data on long-term treatment, Pfizer added open-label extensions to several phase 2 trials, ensuring that regulators would receive data on patients who had been treated for at least a year. Finally, several small-scale RigiScan studies were carried out in which sildenafil was tested and found effective for special populations of ED patients, including men with diabetes and men with spinal cord injuries.[26-28]

Approaching the Finish Line

The phase 2 studies had provided convincing evidence of sildenafil's safety and efficacy. They had also helped the doctors at Pfizer finalize the range of doses—25, 50, and 100 mg—that would be used in the next and pivotal phase of testing: phase 3 studies, which began late in 1995. The phase 3 studies were designed to include the broadest possible range of ED patients, whose clinical characteristics would reflect the population of men who would likely take sildenafil in the "real world" once the drug was released to the market.

"By the time we entered phase 3, we had removed many of the exclusion criteria we had in phase 2," says Dr. Osterloh. "Nevertheless, we very nearly left radical prostatectomy patients out of phase 3

because we thought—mistakenly, as it turns out—that there is no way that sildenafil is going to work for them."

The phase 3 studies included men with ED due to psychogenic causes, men with ED of "mixed" etiology (that is, resulting from both psychogenic and organic causes), and men with ED due to all major organic causes except men with spinal cord injury, who would be studied in a separate large-scale trial.

While men with ED due to nearly all possible etiologies were included in the phase 3 clinical trials, certain exclusionary criteria remained in place throughout these studies. Most importantly, men taking nitrates in any form were excluded (see page 35). Other exclusions were men with serious cardiovascular events within 6 months, uncontrolled hypotension or hypertension, and retinitis pigmentosa.[6] These patients were excluded from the trials because investigators wanted to be confident that subjects were in stable health and not likely to drop out of the trials due to health reasons unrelated to ED. Men with retinitis pigmentosa were excluded because of sildenafil's very modest affinity for PDE 6 in the retina, which led to mild visual side effects in less than 3% of subjects.

"Viagra should be taken about an hour before sexual intercourse, to allow time for maximal absorption of the drug," notes Dr. Peter Ellis of Pfizer Central Research–Sandwich. "But we've done RigiScan studies to find the time interval between taking the drug and when it seems to start working, and that time is 25 minutes. So it's reasonably speedy."

Dr. Ellis continues, "This poses an interesting question for us: Do we need a drug for erectile dysfunction that works faster than 25 minutes after ingestion on an empty stomach? Maybe not. Most people agree that sex is not something to be performed in an instant but rather at your own pace, and that one of the nice things about Viagra is that it allows you time."

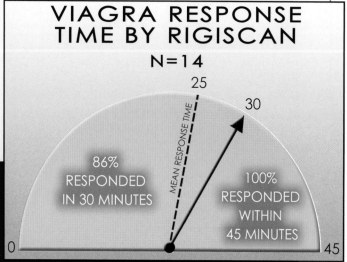

VIAGRA RESPONSE TIME BY RIGISCAN

N=14

86% RESPONDED IN 30 MINUTES

100% RESPONDED WITHIN 45 MINUTES

MEAN RESPONSE TIME

The average time from when subjects swallowed a 50-mg Viagra tablet to onset of erections with sufficient rigidity for sexual intercourse (RigiScan measurement) was shown to be 25 minutes in a study designed to determine the onset and duration of action of Viagra in men with ED. For patients in the Viagra group who responded to the drug, 86% had achieved erections within 30 minutes postdose; the remaining responders had sufficient erections within 45 minutes of ingestion.[6]

Phase 3 began with 4 double-blind, placebo-controlled clinical trials: fixed-dose and flexible-dose trials in the United States, Canada, and Europe. Additional studies were added later, including a study in the United States involving diabetic men with ED. Dr. Pierre Wicker of Pfizer Central Research in Groton, Connecticut, managed the phase 2 and 3 studies in North America.

"Patients and physicians at the research sites were extremely enthusiastic about getting involved, and often we had more patients willing to participate than we could accept in the trials—which is very unusual," observed Dr. Wicker. "With most projects, it is difficult to find patients who qualify and you have to constantly motivate the investigators to recruit for the studies."

A DRUG THAT CAN BE USED WITH OTHERS

Many of the men in the phase 3 trials had concomitant health problems, such as hypertension and diabetes, that required maintenance drug

VIAGRA USE IN SUBJECTS ON MULTIPLE ANTIHYPERTENSIVE DRUGS[6]

TREATMENT RELATED	ANTIHYPERTENSIVE-TREATED PATIENTS	
	On Concomitant Antihypertensive(s) (N=885)	Not on Concomitant Antihypertensive(s) (N=1837)
Syncope	0	0.1%
Dizziness	3.5%	2.3%
Hypotension	0.3%	0.3%
Postural hypotension	0	0.1%

DRUGS TAKEN BY MEN IN VIAGRA CLINICAL TRIALS

WELL TOLERATED IN PATIENTS USING:

✔ Antihypertensives[30]

✔ Antidepressants[6]

✔ Aspirin[6]

✔ Lipid-lowering medications[6]

✔ Antidiabetes drugs[31]

✔ Antacids[6]

✔ Alcohol[6]

treatment. One of the most impressive aspects of sildenafil's safety profile was the paucity of adverse drug events observed in men taking drugs for other health problems at the same time they were taking sildenafil. For example, one third of men enrolled in the clinical trials were also taking at least one antihypertensive medication,[15,29] and they tolerated sildenafil as well as men who were not taking antihypertensives.[30]

ONE NOTABLE EXCEPTION: NITRATES

There is a significant drug interaction with sildenafil, however. As noted in Chapter 2, men taking nitrates in any form—including aerosol, sublingual, or transdermal nitrates—*should not* take sildenafil. The vasodilation from concomitant use of sildenafil and a nitrate can lead to a dangerously abrupt drop in blood pressure.[15] This is stated as a contraindication in the Viagra prescribing information. No men who were taking nitrate medications were included in the clinical trials.

SOME UNDESIRABLE SIDE EFFECTS

As with any drug, Viagra can cause adverse effects. But experience from the clinical trials showed that side effects were generally mild and transient.[30]

MOST COMMONLY RECORDED ADVERSE EVENTS DURING VIAGRA CLINICAL TRIALS[30]

Adverse Effect	Viagra	Placebo
Headache	16%	4%
Flushing	10%	1%
Dyspepsia	7%	2%
Nasal congestion	4%	2%
Abnormal vision*	3%	0%

*Blue tinge or increased light brightness

PATIENTS WANT MORE

"Once a double-blind study finishes, you offer everybody the opportunity to go on the real drug for some period of time afterward—what we call an open-label extension phase of a double-blind study," Dr. Richard Siegel, medical director, Pfizer–New York, explains. "Pfizer Central Research in Groton had been doing that with patients in their double-blind studies. But since the extensions had a defined length of time—1 year—people coming to the end of those open-label studies all of a sudden had to stop taking the drug, and their reactions were not very positive.

"We received a deluge of letters—some were pleading," says Dr. Siegel, recalling one letter in particular: "A man had gotten engaged to be married while he was in the study, and he wrote that his fiancée was threatening to break it off if he stopped taking the medication."

Responding to entreaties from patients, Pfizer extended the open-label extensions for about 1000 phase 2 and 3 patients by an additional 3 years. "That was useful to the patients and to us," says Dr. Siegel, "since we could follow a group of people who were taking the drug for a significant amount of time and be able to get additional information about safety and efficacy."

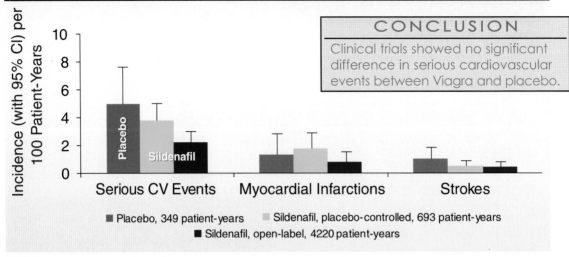

CONCLUSION

Clinical trials showed no significant difference in serious cardiovascular events between Viagra and placebo.

- ■ Placebo, 349 patient-years
- ■ Sildenafil, placebo-controlled, 693 patient-years
- ■ Sildenafil, open-label, 4220 patient-years

As noted in Chapter 2, sildenafil does have transient vasodilatory effects. When complete results of phase 2 and 3 trials were analyzed for adverse events related to lowering of blood pressure, no significant difference was noted between sildenafil and placebo for hypotension, postural hypotension, and syncope. The only significant blood pressure parameter more prevalent in the sildenafil group was dizziness, with 2% of the sildenafil group reporting it versus 1% of the placebo group.[6]

Another way to gauge how well a drug is tolerated is by the number of patients who withdraw from clinical trials. In the Viagra clinical trials, withdrawal was rare and the rate of withdrawal was equivalent in the sildenafil and placebo groups. Of those patients treated with sildenafil, 2.5% withdrew as a result of adverse effects, compared with 2.3% of patients taking the placebo. Headache was the most common adverse effect leading to discontinuation in the trials.[30]

Even men with serious health conditions participated in the clinical trials and tolerated the treatment well. The authors of the *JAMA* article on the use of Viagra in men with diabetes noted,

GLOBAL EFFICACY OF VIAGRA

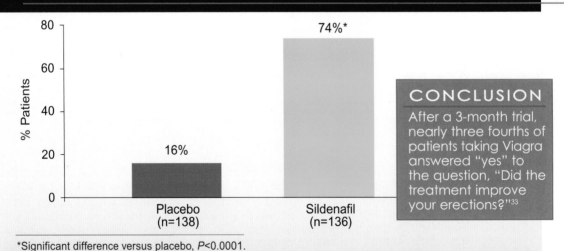

CONCLUSION

After a 3-month trial, nearly three fourths of patients taking Viagra answered "yes" to the question, "Did the treatment improve your erections?"[33]

*Significant difference versus placebo, *P*<0.0001.

This 12-week, double-blind, placebo-controlled study enrolled 329 men with ED of various etiologies. The starting dose was 50 mg, and adjustments to doses of 100 or 25 mg were based on efficacy and tolerability.

"The safety profile of sildenafil in patients with diabetes is reassuring given the chronic complications associated with diabetes."[31]

Throughout the clinical trials, investigators documented all adverse effects, including any cardiovascular effects. When data from the clinical trials were analyzed in terms of patient-years by a team of cardiologists, the incidence of serious cardiovascular effects (including myocardial infarction, angina, and coronary artery disorder) was equivalent in the sildenafil and placebo groups.[32]

A SEND-OFF FOR THE FIRST ORAL ED DRUG

The phase 3 studies had proven eminently successful: Sildenafil had shown itself to have an excellent safety profile while being effective in treating up to 82% of ED patients (compared with 24% of those on placebo) regardless of the cause of their problem.[6] Finally, after 8 years of research and 21 clinical studies in 13 countries involving nearly 4500 men, sildenafil's big day had arrived. **After compiling thousands of pages of clinical data onto a single CD-ROM, Pfizer hand-delivered it to the FDA on September 29, 1997. The Viagra New Drug Application (NDA) had officially been filed.** On the same day, Pfizer officials filed for Viagra approval with the European Medicines Evaluation Agency, which evaluates drugs for the European Union. This was the first time that Pfizer had simultaneously submitted NDAs with 2 large government agencies.

The clinical studies, however, were by no means over. Pfizer would also sponsor an additional 5 phase 3B studies (begun after the NDA was submitted but before the drug was approved) in the United States. These 5 studies were notable for having been carried out by physicians from a variety of specialties.

"Up to that point, almost all the clinical studies in

the US had been done with urologists," says Dr. Richard Siegel, director for medical/sexual health at Pfizer headquarters in New York City, who designed the phase 3B studies. "We knew early on that this drug was going to be prescribed by a lot of physicians other than urologists. So we needed to involve physicians from additional specialties so we could gather data from a broader population of patients."

Four of the 5 phase 3B clinical studies were double-blind, randomized, and placebo-controlled. One, involving men with diabetes who had ED, relied on endocrinologists as investigators. A second study focused on men with concomitant depression and ED and enlisted both urologists and psychiatrists as investigators. A study of men with both multiple sclerosis and ED was conducted by neurologists. The fourth study, which was conducted primarily by urologists, was centered at military medical centers, Veterans Administration hospitals, and HMOs, and enrolled men with ED who had undergone radical prostatectomies. Finally, the fifth phase 3B clinical trial was a large open-label study, which enlisted 75 investigators, 10 of whom were primary care physicians.

VIAGRA SAFETY AND EFFICACY CITED IN MEDICAL LITERATURE

The clinical trials carried out on Viagra have produced a wealth of published studies. This work not only has added greatly to medical knowledge of erectile physiology and ED but has helped make ED an acceptable topic of discussion—between patient and doctor, between men and their partners, and among the public in general. As summed up by an editorial published in *The New England Journal of Medicine* in the same issue as the pivotal US study, **"The availability of sildenafil as an effective and safe oral therapy for men with erectile dysfunction means that**

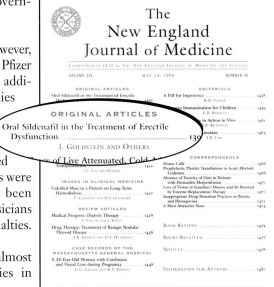

Please see page 85 for a list of selected publications on Viagra, which have appeared in The New England Journal of Medicine, The Lancet, JAMA, Urology, and other well-known medical journals.

many more men will seek help for the condition and that primary care physicians will be increasingly involved in making decisions about the evaluation and treatment of these men."[34]

AN EXTENSIVE— AND IMPRESSIVE— CLINICAL RECORD

The phase 2 and phase 3 studies would involve nearly 4500 men—far more than the average number studied in the course of a typical drug development program. The main reason for the difference: The doctors and executives at Pfizer concluded that they must demonstrate that Viagra worked for ED due to all major causes before they could claim that the medication was an effective treatment for ED. And indeed, Viagra was found to work in all the etiologies for which it was assessed, including cardiovascular disease,[35] diabetes,[31] spinal cord injury,[36] hypertension,[29] post–radical prostatectomy,[37] and depression.[38]

Overall, these clinical studies showed that men with ED who took Viagra experienced significant improvements in erectile function, including a greatly enhanced ability to obtain and maintain an erection and to achieve successful intercourse. ●

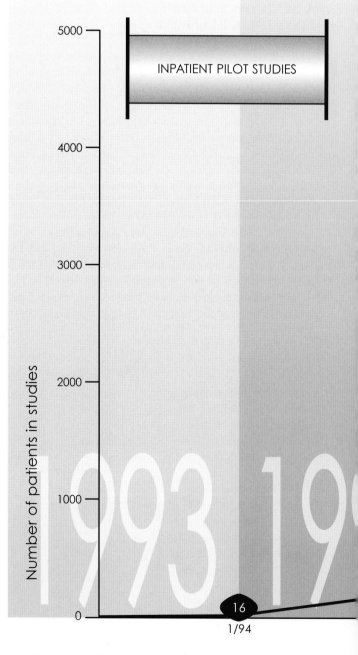

VIAGRA CLINICAL TRIALS TIMELINE

ACCUMULATION OF STUDY SUBJECTS

INPATIENT PILOT STUDIES

Number of patients in studies

1993   19

1/94

16

The Viagra clinical research program started small—enrolling a handful of men with ED who took the drug or placebo in a "laboratory" setting. By the time the clinical trials were completed in early 1997, more than 4000 men had been enrolled.

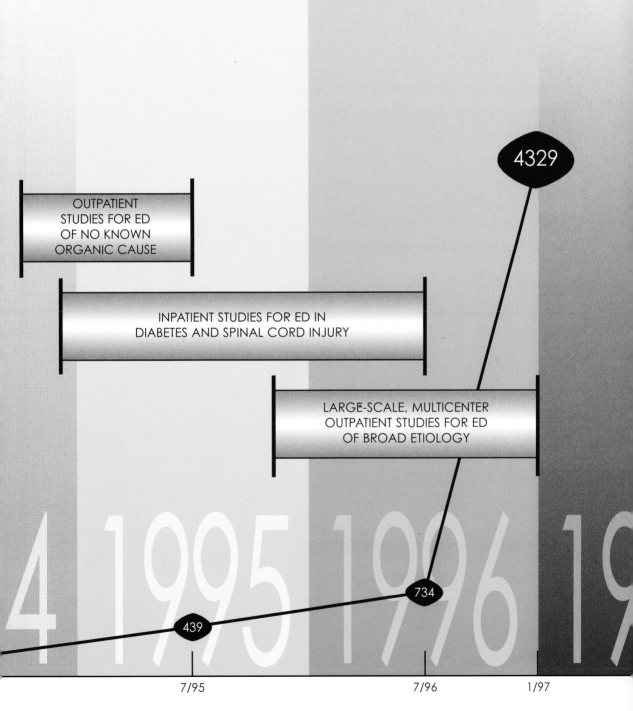

4329

OUTPATIENT STUDIES FOR ED OF NO KNOWN ORGANIC CAUSE

INPATIENT STUDIES FOR ED IN DIABETES AND SPINAL CORD INJURY

LARGE-SCALE, MULTICENTER OUTPATIENT STUDIES FOR ED OF BROAD ETIOLOGY

734

439

7/95   7/96   1/97

Researchers studied Viagra from every possible angle. The following tables depict the ways in which Viagra was measured and found safe and effective:

ETIOLOGY OF ED[39,40]

- ✔ Organic
- ✔ Psychogenic
- ✔ Mixed (organic and psychogenic)

UNDERLYING DISEASE STATE

ETIOLOGY	VIAGRA*
✔ Diabetes[31]	56%
✔ Hypertension[29]	70%
✔ Radical prostatectomy[6]	43%
✔ Spinal cord injury[36]	75%
✔ Ischemic heart disease[35]	70%

*Percentage answering positively to "Did the treatment improve your erections?"

CONCOMITANT MEDICATIONS/DRUGS[6]

STUDIED IN PATIENTS USING:

- ✔ Antihypertensives
- ✔ Antidepressants
- ✔ Aspirin
- ✔ Lipid-lowering medications
- ✔ Antidiabetes drugs
- ✔ Antacids
- ✔ Alcohol

POPULATION SUBGROUPS

- ✔ Coronary artery disease
- ✔ Peripheral vascular disease
- ✔ Diabetes
- ✔ Depression
- ✔ Coronary artery bypass graft
- ✔ Radical prostatectomy
- ✔ Transurethral resection of the prostate
- ✔ Spinal cord injury
- ✔ Hypertension
- ✔ Patients taking antidepressants/antipsychotics
- ✔ Patients taking antihypertensive medications

TRIALS "SCORECARD"

AGE[41]

✔ Under 65   76%*

✔ 65 and over   66%*

*Percentage answering positively to "Did the treatment improve your erections?"

INTERNATIONAL POPULATIONS*

✔ Africa   ✔ Europe

✔ Asia (Japan, China)   ✔ North America

✔ Australia   ✔ South America

*For patients in NDA trials and subsequent studies

ED SEVERITY

✔ Occasional (mild)

✔ Frequent (moderate)

✔ Always (severe)

EFFICACY MEASURES

IMPROVEMENTS IN:

✔ Ability to achieve an erection

✔ Ability to maintain an erection

✔ Quality of erections

✔ IIEF score

✔ Intercourse satisfaction

✔ Orgasmic function

✔ Overall sexual satisfaction

ABOVE OBSERVATION OF IMPROVEMENTS CORROBORATED BY:

✔ Patient diaries

✔ Partner scores

✔ RigiScan measurements

IIEF DOMAIN

IMPROVEMENT IN:

✔ Erectile function

✔ Intercourse satisfaction

✔ Orgasmic function

NOT CLINICALLY SIGNIFICANT ✔ Sexual desire

✔ Overall satisfaction

DURATION OF TREATMENT

PATIENT SATISFACTION AFTER:

✔ 12 weeks[33]   ✔ 1 year[42]

✔ 6 months[40]   ✔ 2 years[43]

REVIEWED AND USED BY MEDICAL SPECIALTIES

✔ Internal medicine

✔ Family practice

✔ Endocrinology

✔ Cardiology

✔ Nephrology

✔ Urology

✔ Psychiatry

✔ Neurology

✔ Oncology

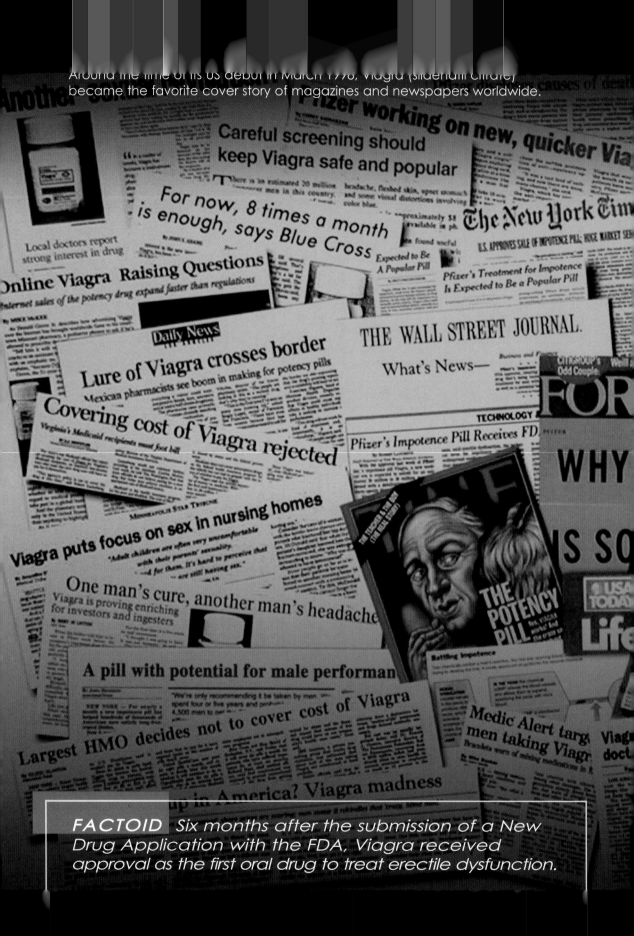

Around the time of its US debut in March 1998, Viagra (sildenafil citrate) became the favorite cover story of magazines and newspapers worldwide.

FACTOID *Six months after the submission of a New Drug Application with the FDA, Viagra received approval as the first oral drug to treat erectile dysfunction.*

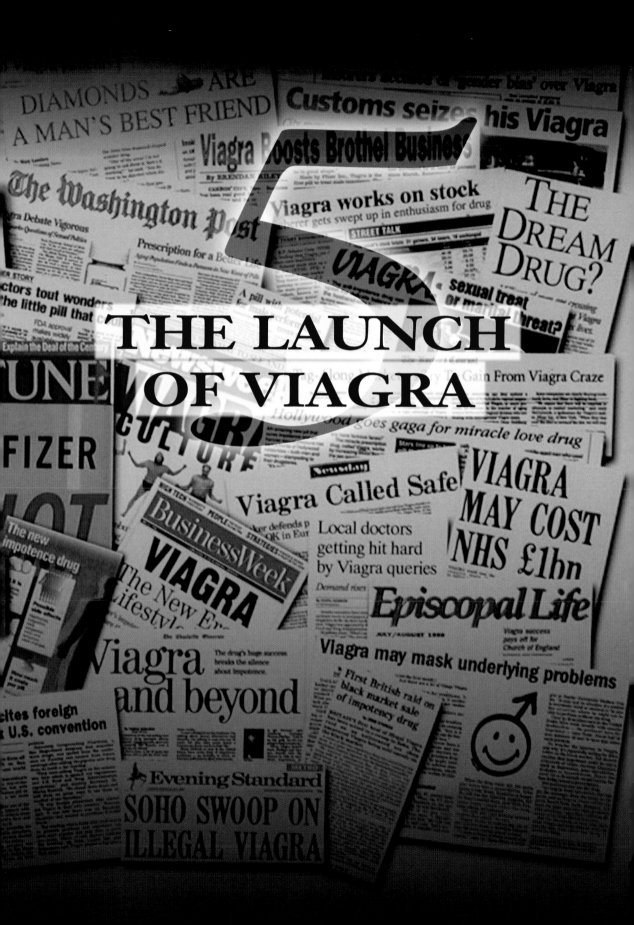

THE LAUNCH
OF VIAGRA

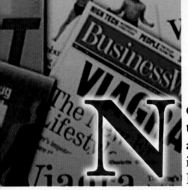

early 10 years of investigation, including 4 years of clinical trials, the combined efforts of hundreds of researchers, and an investment of hundreds of millions of dollars, culminated in a press release issued March 27, 1998: "The Food and Drug Administration today announced the approval of Viagra (sildenafil citrate), the first oral pill to treat impotence, a dysfunction that affects millions of men in the United States."[44]

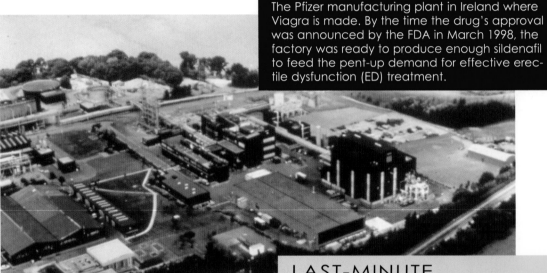

The Pfizer manufacturing plant in Ireland where Viagra is made. By the time the drug's approval was announced by the FDA in March 1998, the factory was ready to produce enough sildenafil to feed the pent-up demand for effective erectile dysfunction (ED) treatment.

FDA APPROVAL IN 6 MONTHS

Pfizer had sent the FDA its New Drug Application for Viagra on September 29, 1997. Three weeks later, the FDA notified Pfizer that it was giving Viagra priority review, which the agency assigns to drugs that fulfill a significant medical need or represent a major advance in therapy.

After the FDA grants priority review, the agency generally responds within 6 months with 1 of 3 actions: a rejection letter, a letter stating that the drug is approvable, or an approval letter.

"We strongly believed, based on the science, that it wasn't going to be rejected, because the drug was unbelievable in clinical trials, just rock-solid," says Dr. Ian Osterloh, medical director, Viagra Team. "The total data package was impressive and one of the best that has ever been submitted."

LAST-MINUTE BUTTERFLIES FOR PFIZER CENTRAL RESEARCH

"We were very confident in the quality of our data and the efficacy and safety of the product. Yet you can never be sure what the regulatory authorities will make of the information you submit. Although the FDA had given Viagra priority-review status and had seemed satisfied with our data and documents at every stage in the review process, some unexpected problems or concerns might still arise. As the deadline for the FDA's decision grew nearer and nearer, the entire team felt increasingly anxious for the final approval.

"When we received the phone call from the FDA that sildenafil would be approved, we felt elation. However, I don't think I ever believed it was definite until our regulatory director went to the FDA to accept the letter of approval personally and then phoned us all at headquarters to tell us that she had it."

Dr. Ian Osterloh, Medical Director, Viagra Team

SOME DRUGS GRANTED PRIORITY FDA REVIEW IN 1998[45]

BRAND NAME	GENERIC NAME	APPROVAL DATE	THERAPEUTIC USE
Refludan	Lepirudin	3-6-98	Heparin-induced thrombocytopenia
Viagra	Sildenafil citrate	3-27-98	Erectile dysfunction
Sucraid	Sacrosidase	4-9-98	Sucrose/isomaltose absorption
Xeloda	Capecitabine	4-30-98	Metastatic breast cancer
Aggrastat	Tirofiban hydrochloride	5-14-98	Unstable angina
Integrilin	Eptifibatide	5-18-98	Anticoagulant for acute coronary syndromes

Viagra joins a select group of drugs that have been given priority review by the FDA, a status granted only to drugs representing a genuine therapeutic breakthrough.

POLLING THE OPINION LEADERS

A year before the launch of Viagra, Pfizer convened a committee of opinion leaders—experts in ethics, sociology, religion, legal issues, urology, cardiology, and female sexuality. Their assignment: Consider the impact that Viagra might have on society and anticipate any unique issues that might arise once Viagra was approved.

"We asked this group to look at the kinds of things that can happen when you start talking about a pill for erectile dysfunction," says David Brinkley, director and worldwide team leader for Viagra. "Do we need to reach out to religious groups that might conclude, 'This is wrong, we shouldn't be helping people have sex?' How will Viagra affect the practice of medicine, and should medical school curricula be revised so that ED and other aspects of sexual health receive more attention? These are the sorts of questions that this group examined with us."

SALES FORCE FACES VIAGRA CHALLENGE

Pfizer also exerted considerable effort in readying its sales force for the debut of Viagra. "We required communications training for the entire sales team—representatives as well as managers," says Hank McCrorie, senior vice president of sales. "Marketing a treatment for ED obviously requires talking about sexual issues, and we wanted to help the sales staff become more comfortable discussing these. And because we anticipated that Viagra might elicit jokes and off-color comments, we had to make sure that our conversations with physicians would remain on a professional level."

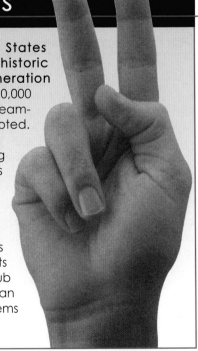

HELLO
MY NAME IS

HOW **VIAGRA**® GOT ITS NAME
(sildenafil citrate) tablets

It's been the subject of endless speculation: Why the name "Viagra"? Was it chosen for its closeness to "vigor"? Or because it sounds like "Niagara," conjuring up images of power, flow, and grandeur? The real explanation is much more mundane. Viagra was chosen mainly for its innocuousness: It was not an English word or a word in any other language and therefore would not cause confusion or embarrassment.

As is typical among pharmaceutical companies, Pfizer works with consultants who create potential drug names, trademark them, and then store them in a "trade names databank." When a new drug needs a brand name, the databank is consulted and candidates are considered.

"A name must satisfy a fairly long list of criteria," says Dr. Pierre Wicker, US team leader for Viagra research at Pfizer Central Research in Groton, Connecticut. "It has to be simple, easy to pronounce, and have no special or unusual meaning in any foreign language. The name goes through a series of linguistic screens and legal screens as well as trademark screens to make sure that no one else is using it." Adds David Brinkley: "We tested it in many different languages to make sure that the meaning was not inappropriate."

To ensure that the appropriate message was delivered to physicians, communications training was supplemented with role-playing. "We had to make sure that our sales team not only understood the product and the medical disorder but knew how to present Viagra appropriately," says Mick Mosebrook, Pfizer group vice president for sales. "We realized we faced skepticism among some doctors about whether ED was even a medical problem. So we needed to convey to doctors not only the importance of treating ED, but the fact that other conditions they treat patients for, such as high blood pressure, may be linked with ED, so it may be worthwhile to ask these patients about their sexual health."

VIAGRA AND BABY BOOMERS

The arrival of Viagra on the scene in the United States coincides with a demographic movement of historic proportions: the transition of the baby boom generation into middle age. Every day, for example, some 10,000 Americans turn 50.[46] Viagra can be viewed as fitting seamlessly into the view of life that baby boomers have adopted.

Unlike previous generations, baby boomers are not willing to regard themselves as middle-aged or resign themselves to the natural shocks that older people are prone to, including ED. Instead, people of this generation want to continue living youthfully and with none of the manifestations of aging that previous generations considered inevitable. Baby boomers are willing to put their efforts where their attitudes are. They are making investments in their health, which may include paying for health-club memberships and new drugs such as Viagra that can manage some of the vexing and common health problems that can occur as they age.

HANDLING THE MEDIA BARRAGE

The approval of Viagra by the FDA touched off a media firestorm that was unprecedented in the history of prescription drugs. Pfizer received word of the approval at 10:57 AM on Friday, March 27, and that afternoon held a press conference featuring Dr. Osterloh and other key investigators. Over the following weeks, the phone calls—from the press, the public, and physicians—flooded in.

The task of handling the media queries fell to Mariann Caprino and Andy McCormick of Pfizer Corporate Communications. "The phone calls were continuous for at least 4 months following approval," says Ms. Caprino.

"We responded to every one and decided early on to be extremely responsive to all media— no matter if it was *The New York Times* or *The Ponca City* [Okla.] *News.*"

Media coverage had actually begun 2 years earlier, when findings

from the Viagra clinical trials were first presented at medical meetings. But it began intensifying in the days preceding approval, with Hugh Downs leading off the March 20 segment of *20/20* with the words, "For the millions of men who want to make love and can't, we are about to make your night." And then, after the approval came the deluge: an outpouring of print and broadcast coverage that would reach some 140 million Americans.[6]

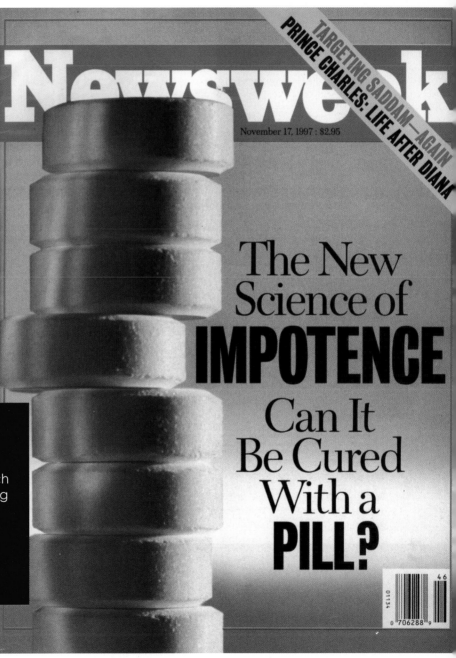

The media hype on Viagra did not begin with its launch after FDA approval in March 1998. It started building in 1997, with a prime example being this cover story in the November 17, 1997, issue of *Newsweek.*

A DRUG UNDER THE MAGNIFYING GLASS

More than most new drugs, Viagra came under intense scrutiny. The media attention lavished on the debut of Viagra soon shifted to possible safety concerns, now that Viagra was being prescribed to hundreds of thousands of men each week. Reports of cardiovascular events and blue-tinted vision among Viagra users captured headlines, as did some predictions that more trouble could lie ahead.

The good news, of course, is that actual experience with Viagra—now prescribed to more than 7 million men in the United States alone[6]—has paralleled the remarkable safety record observed in the clinical trials. And after more than 2 years on the market, it is abundantly clear that Viagra has established a very strong safety record.

REPORTING ADVERSE EVENTS

No clinical trial program, no matter how extensive, can perfectly predict problems that may turn up when a drug goes into general use and is taken by hundreds of thousands of people. Some rare but important adverse drug reactions, for example, may occur at rates of less than 1 in 1000 drug exposures.[47] For this reason, the FDA has developed a postmarketing surveillance effort, called MedWatch, for all drugs, prescription and nonprescription.[47]

Under the agency's MedWatch program, healthcare professionals are asked to report adverse drug events to the agency voluntarily. In fact, any individual, regardless of medical training, can report suspected adverse drug events either to the pharmaceutical company or directly to the FDA. In addition, pharmaceutical companies are required to report such information to the FDA.[47] Pfizer, for its part, has an extensive safety monitoring program and promptly reports adverse events for Viagra and all its other pharmaceuticals—not only to the FDA but to regulatory authorities worldwide.

The MedWatch program is useful but by no means perfect. Adverse-event reports are subjective, may be biased by intense media attention, can vary enormously in quality since they can come from any source—someone's cousin or an ambulance driver, for example—and generally cannot be used to determine either causality or the incidence of a problem. Duplicate reports may occur and are difficult to detect. Because certain health problems, such as myocardial infarction or stroke, occur frequently, it is essentially impossible to determine whether the drug in question caused them. While intense publicity about a certain drug may overestimate the importance or number of reports, problems that occur with other drugs may not be reported and may therefore be underestimated.

Due to the numerous inquiries about Viagra from the press and the public, the FDA took the unprecedented step of posting Viagra-related adverse-event reports on its Web site. Those reports were first posted in June 1998 and were updated the following November.[48]

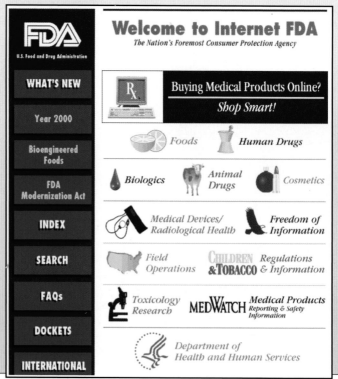

WHAT THE MEDIA SAID ABOUT VIAGRA

CBS EVENING NEWS March 26, 1998 • Dan Rather, anchor

"There could be a major improvement available soon in the medical treatment of impotence. Federal health officials are poised to vote on whether to approve the first potential cure in a pill. CBS's John Roberts reports."

U.S. APPROVES SALE OF IMPOTENCE PILL; HUGE MARKET SEEN

70% of patients helped; eagerly awaited drug found to relieve condition that afflicts millions of men
The New York Times • March 28, 1998 • By Gina Kolata

After months of eager anticipation by patients, doctors and investors, the Food and Drug Administration yesterday approved the first pill for male impotence.

PFIZER'S IMPOTENCE PILL RECEIVES FDA APPROVAL

The Wall Street Journal • March 30, 1998 • By Robert Langreth

With the approval last week of Pfizer Inc.'s impotence pill Viagra, a new medical era is expected to unfold for an estimated 20 million to 30 million men burdened with a debilitating problem few of them openly discuss.

FDA APPROVES FIRST IMPOTENCE PILL

Associated Press • By Lauren Neergaard

Millions of men will soon have access to the first pill to treat impotence, a long-awaited therapy that promises to be easier to use and less embarrassing than traditional treatments.

DOCTORS TOUT WONDERS OF THE LITTLE PILL THAT COULD [lead story]

USA Today • March 29, 1998 • By Tim Friend

The axiom "If it sounds too good to be true, it probably is" often comes to mind when looking at new drug treatments for a disease. But it seems that a little pill called Viagra, approved by the Food and Drug Administration (FDA) on Friday for male impotence, has the USA's leading experts casting aside their usual wait-and-see attitudes.

A REASON FOR HOPE *Los Angeles Times* • March 16, 1998 • By Shari Roan

Every so often, a medication comes along that has the power to change the way a disorder is managed—and to dramatically increase the number of people treated. By most accounts, that is the scenario expected when sildenafil—for the treatment of impotence—is approved by the Food and Drug Administration and reaches the marketplace, probably within months.

PRESCRIPTION FOR LOVE *20/20* • March 20, 1998 • Hugh Downs

"For the millions of men who want to make love and can't, we are about to make your night. An exciting medical breakthrough promises to revolutionize the treatment of sexual impotence. And it could be available in a matter of weeks, because the FDA is expected to approve it very soon."

VIAGRA: IT WORKS!

Viagra tale: How one man sought an impotence cure—& found one
U.S. News & World Report • May 4, 1998 • By Avery Comarow

This is a report from Viagra's front lines. It is from a married man in his early 50s—a friend of this writer who has tried out Pfizer's new impotence drug. Call him X; he does not want his name used. And call him grateful; Viagra worked for him.

A STAMPEDE IS ON FOR IMPOTENCE PILL

The Wall Street Journal • April 20, 1998 • By Robert Langreth and Andrea Petersen

In just two weeks on the market, Pfizer Inc.'s impotence pill Viagra is already one of the fastest-selling drugs in the history of medicine.

ED: JUST ANOTHER LIFESTYLE CHOICE?

"VIAGRA—The New Era of Lifestyle Drugs," proclaimed the cover of Business Week [49] for May 11, 1998. "Pfizer's impotence pill is more than just a blockbuster drug to treat a specific medical problem," the text on the cover continued. "It will also enhance the quality of life for 'healthy' people." Featured front and center on the cover: a round tablet with a smiley face inscribed.

It was just one of many press reports that have dubbed Viagra a "lifestyle" drug, a "performance-enhancing" drug, or a drug for improving "quality of life."

Many reports on the lifestyle aspect go on to say that Viagra doesn't deserve the status—or the insurance reimbursement—reserved for drugs that address more "serious" health problems.

Less than 2 months after the approval of Viagra, for example, an article in the Atlanta Journal and Constitution stated that "many managed care companies are questioning whether drugs that enhance a patient's quality of life—such as Viagra—should be covered with the same consistency as pills that treat life-threatening conditions, such as heart disease or cancer."[50]

These articles reveal a basic misunderstanding of ED, suggesting it is more of a lifestyle choice (like choosing abstinence) than a medical condition. Reflecting the view that prevailed 30 years ago, such articles often portray ED as mainly an emotional hang-up.

"The impotence drug Viagra, which offers erection-in-a-pill, has taken the country by storm," wrote The Gazette of Montreal. "Sex therapists have been telling us for years: When it comes to sex, the mind and emotions are as important as the plumbing. The message for men? Relax. Take a deep breath. Don't rush. You might save yourself 10 bucks."[51]

If only it were that easy. It's now known that some 80% of ED cases stem from physical problems that affect the vessels or nerves, such as atherosclerosis or diabetes.[2] And for the 20% of men whose ED results from anxiety or some other psychological problem: Try telling them that their anguish is less intense than if their problem had arisen from a physical cause!

"VIAGRA" BECOMES A FAMILIAR NAME

"It would have been hard to predict how quickly Viagra got into the public discourse," says Mr. Brinkley. "Before approval, we used to wonder, 'Gee, I wonder if Jay Leno will ever make a joke about Viagra.' And then, of course, he ended up telling a Viagra joke every night for weeks."

In a matter of weeks, awareness of Viagra achieved levels usually reserved for long-established products like Coke or Pepsi, with more than 90% of American adults able to recognize the name.

A HIT WITH DOCTORS AND PATIENTS

The instant fame of Viagra was paralleled by its rapid acceptance by the medical community and men with ED. Before Viagra, less than 10% of men with ED had sought medical help for their problem.[6] But Viagra finally gave them a reason to seek treatment. And seek it they did: Physicians wrote 5.3 million prescriptions for Viagra during its first 6 months on the market, the most successful introduction ever for a US drug at that time.[6]

The New England Journal of Medicine, May 14, 1998

A Pill for Impotence

"In this issue of the Journal, Goldstein et al. describe the efficacy of oral sildenafil in men with erectile dysfunction. . . . The results of this study are promising, and the drug has been widely hailed in the media since its approval by the Food and Drug Administration on March 27. Anecdotes of nearly miraculous restoration of sexual function have fueled the excitement. . . ."[34]

—Robert D. Utiger, MD

Geriatrics, October 10, 1998

The Viagra Revolution: Drug for erectile dysfunction is redefining our ideas about sexuality among older couples

"Thirty-five years ago 'The Pill' sparked a sexual revolution among the young. In 1998, sildenafil citrate (Viagra) may be instigating another sexual revolution, this time among persons middle-aged and older. . . . Viagra is neither an aphrodisiac nor a love potion for relationships in distress. It is a vehicle that can help couples enjoy the pleasures of sex and circumvent the disabling, demoralizing effects of erectile dysfunction."[53]

—Robert N. Butler, MD

British Medical Journal, September 19, 1998

Viagra: on release. Evidence on the effectiveness of sildenafil is good.

"The popular interest in Viagra (sildenafil) is not solely the result of media hype and the drug's association with sex: the demand for treatment has been enormous. . . . The level of demand was predictable, given a prevalence of erectile dysfunction of over 50% in men aged 50–70, and the unacceptability, poor effectiveness, or unavailability of existing treatments. . . . To most sufferers, a tablet treatment must have seemed too good to be true. A localized effect after oral administration is possible because of sildenafil's specificity of action. . . ."[52]

—Alain Gregoire, MD

BOB DOLE BECOMES ED SPOKESMAN

Former US Senator and presidential candidate Bob Dole was one of the radical prostatectomy patients enrolled in the Viagra clinical trials. He revealed his participation on *Larry King Live* in May 1998, shortly after Viagra was approved, endorsing it as "a great drug." A few days later, Elizabeth Dole echoed her husband's verdict by describing Viagra as "a great drug."

So it was perhaps only natural that Bob Dole agreed to participate with Pfizer in an educational initiative designed to increase public awareness of men's health issues, including ED. **"I'm convinced this campaign can help promote a dialogue between doctors and patients and help men pay attention to health problems they might otherwise be afraid to discuss,"** Mr. Dole said on assuming his new role.

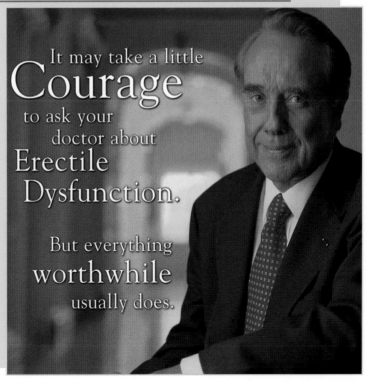

It may take a little **Courage** to ask your doctor about **Erectile Dysfunction.**

But everything **worthwhile** usually does.

VIEW FROM A PRIMARY CARE PHYSICIAN

Dr. Richard Sadovsky, a primary care physician and faculty member in the Family Practice Department at State University of New York Health Science Center, Brooklyn, New York, comments on how he sees the effect of Viagra on primary care:

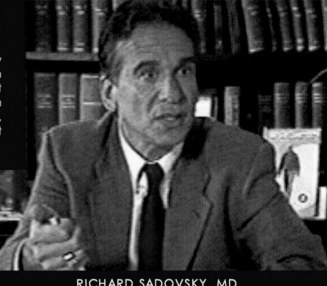

RICHARD SADOVSKY, MD

In the pre-Viagra era, I asked patients about their sexual activity to see if unsafe practices were putting them at risk of infections such as HIV or hepatitis. But now that Viagra is available, I've added questions to the sexual history that involve sexual function and satisfaction—specifically, "Are you satisfied with sex?"

I've found that patients are very willing and receptive to discussing sexual satisfaction and are actually happy when I introduce the topic. These conversations have even helped to improve my clinical relationship with patients, allowing them to discuss their feelings about other issues more easily. **However, many primary care physicians have yet to see the effects of Viagra in their practice because they steer clear of discussing sex.**

Primary care physicians are under great pressure to do everything and do it efficiently. Their main priorities are diseases that have high morbidity and mortality or are disabling. So doctors may tend to overlook ED because they don't see it as a problem that causes morbidity.

Instead, doctors see ED as a quality-of-life issue, and a lot of doctors feel that they're not supposed to get involved with those issues any more than they should get involved with the quality of a patient's sofa: It just isn't necessary, and we have so much else to do that there just isn't time. But a survey published in February 1999 in *JAMA* may help to counter that assumption.

The National Health and Social Life Survey looked at the prevalence of sexual dysfunction among American men and women aged 18 to 59. Sexual problems were found to affect over 30% of men and more than 40% of women.[54] This and other surveys have found that ED is associated with morbidities of its own, including anxiety, depression, decreased self-esteem, difficulty with relationships, and a generally diminished quality of life.[54]

This survey has given me a chance to tell my associates, **"You know, 1 out of 3 18- to 59-year-old men who walks into your office has some dissatisfaction with sexual activity, and dissatisfaction is probably even more prevalent among older men, since the likelihood of ED increases with age."** So it's really a very common problem.

I've treated about 30 patients with Viagra. Based on reports from patients, it appears that the drug has been successful about 80% of the time. **Being able to alleviate ED—a problem that has such a major impact on patients' lives—has made practicing medicine more rewarding for me. Not only are patients happy but the intervention itself—prescribing Viagra—is simple to do, usually effective, and in my experience quite safe.**

As a testament to the effectiveness of Viagra, approximately 50% of all Viagra prescriptions are refills.[6] And as a testament to its ability to get men to see their doctors, 6 million of the estimated 30 million American men with ED received prescriptions in the first 18 months Viagra was on the market.[6]

Many health insurance plans are not willing to reimburse men for the cost of Viagra prescriptions. Yet Viagra has become so well accepted that a large percentage of patients are willing to pay for it out of their own pockets.

PRIMARY CARE PHYSICIANS: THE FRONT LINE OF TREATMENT

So far, more than 300,000 physicians have prescribed Viagra for approximately 7 million men with ED in the United States. The doctors most responsible for handling this surge of patients—who have written 60% of all prescriptions for Viagra—are primary care physicians.[6]

SITUATION WORLDWIDE

Less than 2 years after the approval of Viagra in the United States, the drug had been approved in 99 countries. Worldwide, some 10 million Viagra tablets are now being dispensed each month, and sales exceeded $1 billion within 5 months of the launch. Viagra has captured more than 90% of the market for male ED treatments.[6] ●

VIAGRA AND PRIMARY CARE: A POSITIVE COMBINATION

"So much of what doctors do to manage their patients' health amounts to haranguing them to do things that detract from their enjoyment of life—saying things like, 'You really should lose some weight,' or, 'You've got to stop smoking,' or, 'Cut down on salty and fatty foods.'

"That's particularly true for primary care physicians, because we're on the frontlines for handling chronic problems such as obesity, hypertension, and diabetes," comments Dr. Richard Sadovsky. "Viagra offers an easy way for us to make a huge difference in our patients' lives by giving them something, rather than taking things away."

VIAGRA RECOGNITION NEAR AND FAR

The 1999 *Oxford Dictionary of New Words* lists "Viagra"—record time for any product from time of introduction to time of inclusion in a dictionary.

At least 19 consumer books about Viagra have been published since its approval.

On a recent trip to Kyrgyzstan, a remote country that was part of the former Soviet Union, a visitor saw just 2 recognizable signs in the streets of Bishkek, the capital: "Stop" and "Viagra."

The popular Brazilian magazine *Veja* featured an article on "A Pílula Milagrosa" (The Miracle Pill)

Cyberspace phenomenon: Web sites on Viagra sprang up seemingly overnight. One count in November 1999 revealed 48 sites offering advice, tales of personal experience, and even live chat rooms.

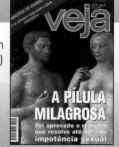

VIAGRA (sildenafil citrate) WORLDWIDE AVAILABILITY

It's a Viagra world. As of the end of 1999, 99 countries had approved the erection drug and 77 had launched the sale of Viagra. Dates listed are the official launch dates for each country in which Viagra is sold.[6]

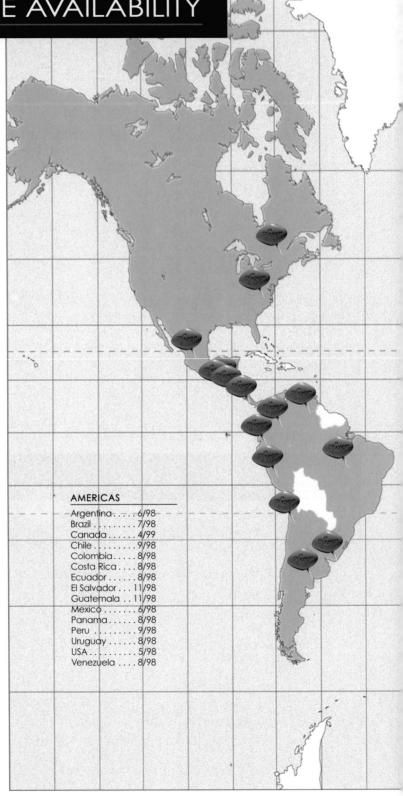

AMERICAS

Argentina 6/98
Brazil 7/98
Canada 4/99
Chile 9/98
Colombia 8/98
Costa Rica 8/98
Ecuador 8/98
El Salvador . . . 11/98
Guatemala . . 11/98
Mexico 6/98
Panama 8/98
Peru 9/98
Uruguay 8/98
USA 5/98
Venezuela 8/98

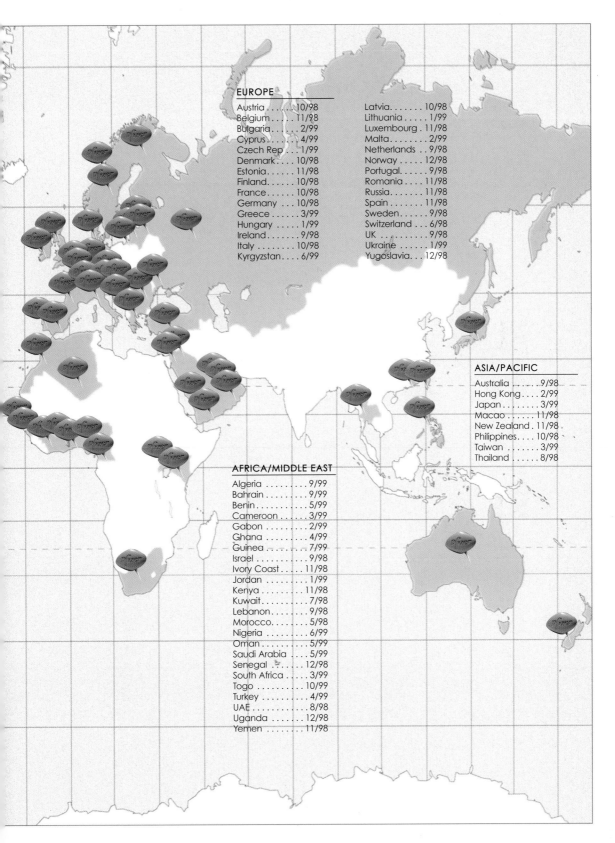

EUROPE

Austria	10/98	Latvia	10/98
Belgium	11/98	Lithuania	1/99
Bulgaria	2/99	Luxembourg	11/98
Cyprus	4/99	Malta	2/99
Czech Rep	1/99	Netherlands	9/98
Denmark	10/98	Norway	12/98
Estonia	11/98	Portugal	9/98
Finland	10/98	Romania	11/98
France	10/98	Russia	11/98
Germany	10/98	Spain	11/98
Greece	3/99	Sweden	9/98
Hungary	1/99	Switzerland	6/98
Ireland	9/98	UK	9/98
Italy	10/98	Ukraine	1/99
Kyrgyzstan	6/99	Yugoslavia	12/98

ASIA/PACIFIC

Australia	9/98
Hong Kong	2/99
Japan	3/99
Macao	11/98
New Zealand	11/98
Philippines	10/98
Taiwan	3/99
Thailand	8/98

AFRICA/MIDDLE EAST

Algeria	9/99
Bahrain	9/99
Benin	5/99
Cameroon	3/99
Gabon	2/99
Ghana	4/99
Guinea	7/99
Israel	9/98
Ivory Coast	11/98
Jordan	1/99
Kenya	11/98
Kuwait	7/98
Lebanon	9/98
Morocco	5/98
Nigeria	6/99
Oman	5/99
Saudi Arabia	5/99
Senegal	12/98
South Africa	3/99
Togo	10/99
Turkey	4/99
UAE	8/98
Uganda	12/98
Yemen	11/98

While Viagra (sildenafil citrate) is a "new millennium" drug for an age-old disorder—erectile dysfunction—diagnosing this disorder is very "low tech." It's primarily a matter of asking the right questions—and asking them of the right patients, since all men over 40 are at risk for erectile dysfunction.

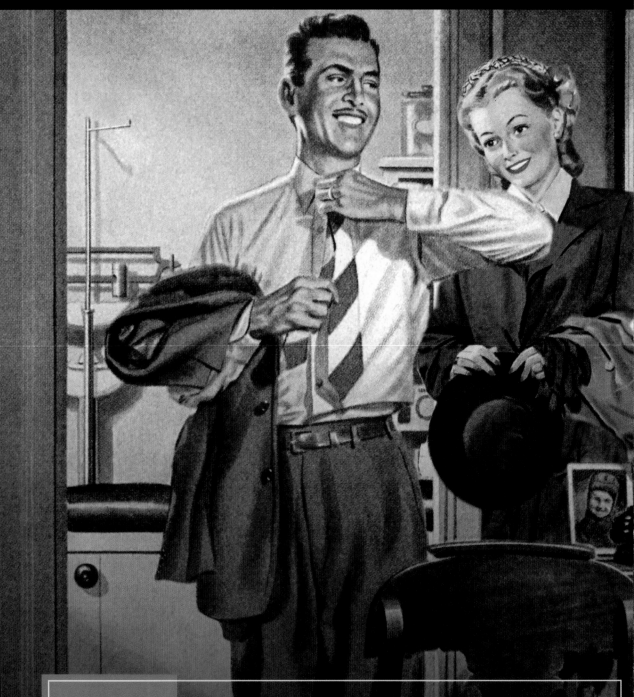

FACTOID *Physicians wrote 5.3 million prescriptions for Viagra during its first 6 months on the market—making Viagra at that time the most successful introduction ever for a US pharmaceutical.*

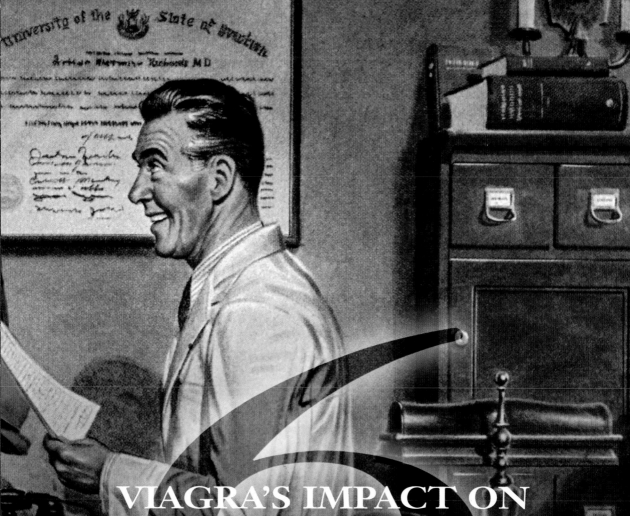

VIAGRA'S IMPACT ON THE DIAGNOSIS AND TREATMENT OF ERECTILE DYSFUNCTION

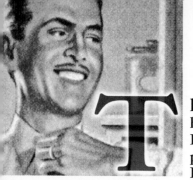

The main obstacle to diagnosing erectile dysfunction (ED) has nothing to do with lack of medical knowledge or technology. It is the "don't ask, don't tell" policy that often prevails between patient and doctor when it comes to discussing sexual health. Patients are frequently too embarrassed to reveal they have a problem. So it's often up to the doctor to broach the subject. But doctors may be hesitant to ask patients about their sex lives, and such questions are not yet a routine part of the medical history. Fortunately, Viagra (sildenafil citrate) is making it easier for doctors and patients to have that conversation about sex, which can have significance far beyond ED itself.

VIAGRA BRINGS ABOUT A CHANGE IN ATTITUDE

Today, men undergoing a routine exam may be more willing to raise the issue of ED on their own, since most of them have heard of Viagra and may hope it will work for them. And since Viagra's highly publicized launch, more men than ever are making appointments to see their doctors specifically about ED treatment. As of June 2000, Viagra had been prescribed to 7 million men in the United States.[6] Despite men's awareness, however, in most cases the physician will need to take the initiative in discussing a patient's sexual history, which means posing some carefully phrased questions about lifestyle choices and health problems.

ASKING THE RIGHT QUESTIONS

Successful questioning should uncover the patient's specific complaint as well as the details of his ED. These details should include an attempt to pinpoint when the ED started and how often it has occurred. Ideally, the questions should not seem intrusive.

"I use two sets of questions," offers Dr. Richard Sadovsky, a primary care physician in Brooklyn, New York. "The first is for patients with an identifiable risk factor associated with ED, such

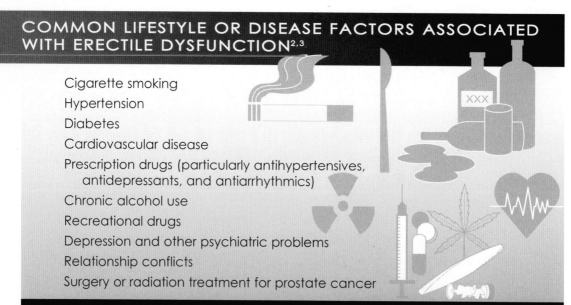

COMMON LIFESTYLE OR DISEASE FACTORS ASSOCIATED WITH ERECTILE DYSFUNCTION[2,3]

Cigarette smoking

Hypertension

Diabetes

Cardiovascular disease

Prescription drugs (particularly antihypertensives, antidepressants, and antiarrhythmics)

Chronic alcohol use

Recreational drugs

Depression and other psychiatric problems

Relationship conflicts

Surgery or radiation treatment for prostate cancer

Men with one or more of the above lifestyle or disease factors are more likely to have ED.

as smoking, hypertension, or diabetes. The objective here is to make sure the patient won't feel unique. So for smokers I would say, 'Many of my male patients who smoke seem to be having difficulty with erections—how about you?' That way, I tell them I've heard this from other patients and I won't be surprised if they say yes.

"For patients who don't have apparent risk factors for ED but are over 40, the questions start out general in nature and then get more precise as the patient provides information," says Dr. Sadovsky. "I say, 'It's important for me to talk to you a little bit about your sexual activity because it may increase your risk for infectious diseases or indicate a more serious underlying condition. Can you tell me a little bit about your sexual activity?' I then try to find out who their partners are, what they're doing, whether they're enjoying it, and whether they're satisfied, reminding them that this is all confidential.

"When I ultimately start asking about ED—'How long has it been since you've had an erection?' for example—you'd expect some patients would say, 'I don't want to talk about it.' But I've never actually had that happen—ever. I think it's crystal clear that patients are more willing to talk about sex than their physicians are. But the doctor often has to get the conversation going."

WHAT THE SURVEYS SHOW

Two recent national surveys have shed light on attitudes towards ED and Viagra. The National Men's Health Week Survey, carried out by *Men's Health* magazine and CNN and released in June 1999, found that Viagra may have made some men more willing to see physicians for ED. However, 37% of those surveyed said they would hesitate in seeking treatment even if they had symptoms of ED. Also, 26% of the men surveyed said they would wait a month or more before seeking treatment; 11% would not see a doctor at all if they thought they might need Viagra.[55]

The second survey, sponsored by AARP and *Modern Maturity* magazine, assessed the sexual attitudes and practices of American men and women aged 45 and older. The survey, released in 1999, found that only 2.5% of men under 60 had complete ED, but the figure rose to almost 16% for those 60 through 74.[56] A total of 5.6% of the men surveyed (about 25% of those with some degree of ED) said they were currently using a treatment to enhance sexual performance,[57] with half of those under treatment using Viagra. A majority of men using Viagra or other medical intervention and a majority of women whose partners were being tested said the drug had increased their enjoyment of sex. *Modern Maturity* provided an anecdote from one woman in her mid-50s who said this about her spouse's use of Viagra: "It was a wonderful feeling to be satisfied again."[56]

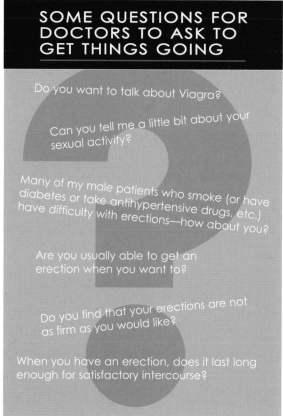

SOME QUESTIONS FOR DOCTORS TO ASK TO GET THINGS GOING

Do you want to talk about Viagra?

Can you tell me a little bit about your sexual activity?

Many of my male patients who smoke (or have diabetes or take antihypertensive drugs, etc.) have difficulty with erections—how about you?

Are you usually able to get an erection when you want to?

Do you find that your erections are not as firm as you would like?

When you have an erection, does it last long enough for satisfactory intercourse?

ED ENTERS THE PRIMARY CARE REALM

Until Viagra's arrival, ED was considered primarily a subspecialty of urology. Shortly after Viagra's launch, urologists themselves heralded a change. "The availability of sildenafil, the first effective oral agent for ED, has expanded the field of sexual healthcare to include general and primary care practitioners and other non-urology specialists," notes

The comments of Dr. Richard Sadovsky, a primary care physician in Brooklyn, New York, illustrate how ED is evolving from a forbidden topic to a condition that primary care physicians are becoming more confident in diagnosing and treating.

I've always thought it's very important to take sexual histories, in part to evaluate patients' risks for HIV and hepatitis B and C. This was a standard part of my patient history for all my patients. Unfortunately, very few doctors have been willing to do that.

Many have felt it would be mutually embarrassing. Or they felt that asking patients about sex may open a Pandora's box they wouldn't be able to close, particularly if patients told them about sexual activities that made them uncomfortable, were risky, or were evidence of some kind of sexual dysfunction. **Sex and ED were seen as the realm of the urologist or gynecologist. And since very few patients actually brought it up, the general practitioner was very happy not to talk about it at all.**

Then along came Viagra, which brought a certain number of ED patients who had never sought help out of the woodwork and into our offices. But primary care physicians still felt that sexual activity was a difficult topic to bring up. And since we have so many guidelines to meet and so much preventive healthcare to do, there just wasn't a lot of time to discuss the subject.

Not long after Viagra's approval, reports of cardiac deaths alleged to be associated with its use received a lot of press attention. That scared many primary care doctors, especially since many of the patients who have ED also have cardiovascular disease.

I sometimes ask my audience at primary care meetings, "How many of you are concerned about the cardiac side effects of sildenafil citrate?" Every single doctor has raised his or her hands. I think a lot of them had adopted a wait-and-see attitude, partly because primary care doctors typically don't use new drugs when they first come out. Instead, they like to hear about the experiences that subspecialists have had before prescribing a drug themselves.

We, as primary care physicians, often clear our patients for surgery—a big responsibility, but we do so because we deem it necessary. But to clear patients to take Viagra seemed like more of a risk, since we regard ED more as a lifestyle issue than as a health problem that required treatment. So the possibility of cardiac problems with Viagra was another reason—an excuse, actually—for doctors not to ask patients about sexual dysfunction.

Primary care physicians hesitate to deal with ED because they want to know, "What are we trying to obtain with treatment?" "What is the goal of treatment?" That's why it's helpful to look at articles by Dr. Tom Lue, a urologist who writes about goal-oriented treatment for ED.[58] Goal-oriented treatment is something that we know about in primary care, but we aren't familiar with the goals in treating ED.

The number-one goal is to help your patients have better erections, pure and simple. Number two is to help them have more satisfying sexual relations. And number three is improving their relationships with whomever they're close to. So it starts to become clearer that ED treatment involves more than just restoring a person's ability to have an erection.

I think there's an analogy to be drawn between primary care physicians treating sexual dysfunction and treating depression. Even when antidepressants were introduced that were safe and easy to use—the SSRIs—primary care doctors still didn't want to determine which of their patients were depressed and offered a lot of reasons for not doing so: "What a ball of wax it'll be," "What am I supposed to do?" "I don't know much about the medication," "It takes too much time," " I don't know how to do the counseling."

But now, primary care physicians are routinely treating depression, and depression really has become a disease with a primary care focus. So I would wager that ED is going to become more of a primary care disease in the future. I think it's going to be a 3- to 5-year evolution before primary care doctors realize that ED has morbidity associated with it and that there's a treatment with an excellent safety profile that doesn't require a lot of their time.

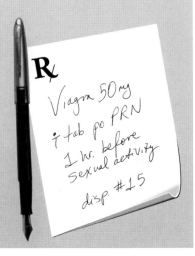

SELF-RATING OF ERECTILE FUNCTION:

These questions make up the Sexual Health Inventory for Men (SHIM), a validated, abridged version of the IIEF that patients can fill out to help determine if they have erectile dysfunction. Men who score 21 or less are advised to speak to their doctors.

Over the past 6 months:

1. How do you rate your *confidence* that you could get and keep an erection?

Very low	Low	Moderate	High	Very high
1	2	3	4	5

2. When you had erections with sexual stimulation, *how often* were your erections hard enough for penetration (entering your partner)?

No sexual activity	Almost never or never	A few times (much less than half the time)	Sometimes (about half the time)	Most times (much more than half the time)	Almost always or always
0	1	2	3	4	5

3. During sexual intercourse, *how often* were you able to maintain your erection after you had penetrated (entered) your partner?

Did not attempt intercourse	Almost never or never	A few times (much less than half the time)	Sometimes (about half the time)	Most times (much more than half the time)	Almost always or always
0	1	2	3	4	5

4. During sexual intercourse, *how difficult* was it to maintain your erection to completion of intercourse?

Did not attempt intercourse	Extremely difficult	Very difficult	Difficult	Slightly difficult	Not difficult
0	1	2	3	4	5

5. When you attempted sexual intercourse, *how often* was it satisfactory for you?

Did not attempt intercourse	Almost never or never	A few times (much less than half the time)	Sometimes (about half the time)	Most times (much more than half the time)	Almost always or always
0	1	2	3	4	5

INTERPRETING THE SHIM

No ED:	22–25
Mild ED:	17–21
Mild to moderate ED:	12–16
Moderate ED:	8–11
Severe ED:	1–7

Dr. Harin Padma-Nathan, a urologist and director of the Male Clinic in Beverly Hills, California.[59]

By late 1999, 60% of all Viagra prescriptions were being written by primary care physicians[6]: clear evidence that ED treatment has abruptly expanded from a specialist concern to a primary care issue.

TRANSFORMING A RESEARCH INSTRUMENT INTO A PRACTICAL DIAGNOSTIC TOOL

After interviewing primary care physicians and urologists, Pfizer researchers realized that an abridged version of the 15-item IIEF questionnaire (see page 29)—later to become the 5-question Sexual Health Inventory for Men (SHIM)[60]— would be more acceptable to both doctors and patients for diagnosing men with ED and for

In patients reporting ED, the physical exam may include many of the same components that are done routinely. It includes a cardiovascular exam, a neurologic exam, an evaluation for gynecomastia and secondary male sexual characteristics, a genital exam (looking for penile abnormalities and examining the testicles for size and consistency), and a digital rectal exam to evaluate the prostate.[3]

ED can usually be diagnosed without extensive tests. Nevertheless, according to the NIH Panel on Impotence, certain laboratory tests for men with ED may be indicated, since they may reveal abnormalities that contribute to ED.[3] Low serum testosterone levels, for example, are rarely the sole cause of ED, but diminished libido caused by low testosterone may play a role. Other lab tests—complete blood count, urinalysis, serum creatinine and blood glucose levels, lipid profile, and thyroid function studies—may implicate previously unrecognized systemic diseases, such as diabetes or heart disease, that are the underlying cause of ED.[3]

facilitating doctor-patient communication about the problem.

"Erectile dysfunction is a very sensitive topic, and our research determined that an easy-to-use, robust, and accurate instrument could aid in diagnosing the condition," says Dr. Joseph C. Cappelleri, associate director of biometrics in the statistics group at Pfizer Central Research in Groton, Connecticut. "We constructed the SHIM by selecting the 5 questions from the 15-question IIEF that could best discriminate between the presence and absence of ED while conforming to the National Institutes of Health definition of ED."

Dr. Cappelleri and his colleagues then evaluated the SHIM—pulling answers to the 5 SHIM questions from more than 1000 IIEF questionnaires filled out by men with diagnosed ED in the Viagra clinical trials and by men without diagnosed ED from outpatient clinics. "The data suggest that the SHIM is an excellent diagnostic tool for discriminating between men with and men without

PRESCRIPTION DRUGS SOMETIMES ASSOCIATED WITH ED[61]

H₂ receptor blockers

Ketoconazole

Antidepressants

Antihypertensives
  – Beta blockers
  – Diuretics

Phenothiazines

Lipid-lowering agents

Cytotoxics

Antiandrogens

For patients who have ED and who are taking one or more of the above prescription drugs, trying a lower dose or switching to a different medication may help to alleviate their ED, as long as this can be done without jeopardizing the efficacy of the treatment for which the drug was prescribed.

ED and for determining the severity of ED," says Dr. Cappelleri.

The SHIM asks men to respond to 5 specific questions about sexual functioning over the previous 6 months. Four of the questions have a scale from 0 to 5, with 0 indicating no activity; the fifth question—"How do you rate your confidence that you could get and keep an erection?"—has a scale of 1 to 5, with 1 signifying "very low." SHIM scores can range from 1 to 25, with scores 22 and above indicating normal erectile function and scores of 11 and below suggesting moderate to severe erectile dysfunction.[58] When administering the SHIM, physicians should ask patients about their desire and opportunity for sexual activity to ensure that low scores are truly indicative of severe ED.

VIAGRA-INSPIRED ED CHECKUPS SAVE LIVES

Thanks to the publicity surrounding Viagra, more men are going to see a doctor—and many of these men may be saving their

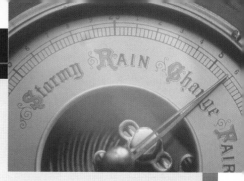

A crucial reason for questioning men about ED is that it may be an early sign of an underlying and potentially serious health condition. For example, up to 15% of apparently healthy men presenting with ED have abnormal glucose tolerance.[2]

Diabetes is just one serious condition that can be signaled by ED. Diagnosing ED can also be lifesaving if it leads to the detection and treatment of underlying heart disease. Atherosclerotic disease is the most common cause of organic ED, accounting for nearly 50% of all cases in men over age 50.[61] As illustrated by a recent study, ED may be one of the first symptoms of cardiovascular disease, since the narrow vessels of the penis appear to be more sensitive to atherosclerotic blockage than the larger vessels of the heart.

Researchers at the Minneapolis Heart Institute Foundation reviewed the histories and test results of 50 men with ED who had sought prescriptions for Viagra and were referred by their physicians for further evaluation. While none of the men had symptoms of heart disease, 20 of them, or 40%, were found to have significant blockages in their coronary arteries. The study was reported in November 1999 at the American Heart Association Scientific Sessions in Atlanta.[62]

"Erectile dysfunction could be called a 'penile stress test,' and may be another way for detecting diseased blood vessels," says Dr. Marc R. Pritzker of the Minneapolis Heart Institute Foundation. He noted that Viagra, by bringing men with ED into doctors' offices, has significant implications for public health. "We now have another opportunity to look for heart disease, make a diagnosis, and offer appropriate prevention and, if necessary, treatment to men in an age group at risk for vascular disease who often don't visit a physician for routine checkups." Only 15 of the 50 men in the study had seen a physician within the 2 years before seeking treatment for ED.[62]

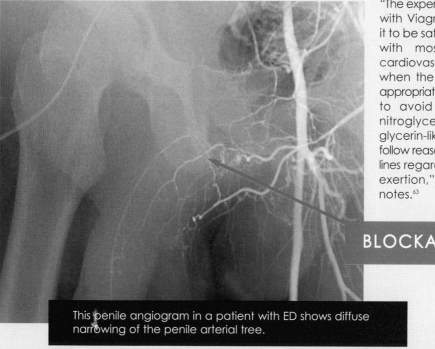

"The experience to date with Viagra has shown it to be safe for patients with most forms of cardiovascular disease when the patients are appropriately counseled to avoid the use of nitroglycerin or nitro-glycerin-like drugs and follow reasonable guidelines regarding physical exertion," Dr. Pritzker notes.[63]

BLOCKAGE

This penile angiogram in a patient with ED shows diffuse narrowing of the penile arterial tree.

lives by doing so. A study presented at the 1999 annual meeting of the American Urological Association demonstrated that evaluating men with ED can reveal previously unrecognized malignancies. Over the course of 1 year (July 1, 1997, to July 1, 1998), urologists in Winston-Salem, North Carolina, thoroughly evaluated 207 new patients with a mean age of 60 years who presented solely with the complaint of erectile dysfunction. Thirty-one of these 207 men—15%—ultimately were diagnosed with urologic malignancies: 16 were found to have prostate cancer, 12 had transitional cell carcinoma of the bladder, 2 were diagnosed with renal cell carcinoma, and 1 was found to have squamous cell carcinoma of the penis.[64]

Cancer is not the only life-threatening condition that may be first diagnosed after the appearance of ED. Coronary artery disease is another. Researchers at the Minneapolis Heart Institute Foundation found that 40% of men seeking prescriptions for Viagra had significant atherosclerosis.[62] (See ED as a Health "Barometer" on page 63.)

FROM DIAGNOSIS TO TREATMENT: A STEP-BY-STEP PROCESS

Once a diagnosis of ED has been established—through history-taking, physical exam, laboratory tests, or some combination—it is often useful to look for underlying causes before beginning ED treatment, since ED is usually a symptom of one or more health conditions. Correcting the underlying problem—if possible—may therefore be the best course of action, not only for treating ED but for the patient's overall health as well.

Unfortunately, the root causes of ED—penile vessels damaged by atherosclerosis, for example, or nerve damage due to diabetes—usually cannot be reversed. So as a practical matter, treatment for ED is usually directed at the penis, through treatment techniques including Viagra, vacuum constriction devices, or penile injections. Studies have shown that the underlying cause of ED rarely influences the choice of therapy.[65] Furthermore, in many cases, physicians may not be able to determine the precise cause of the

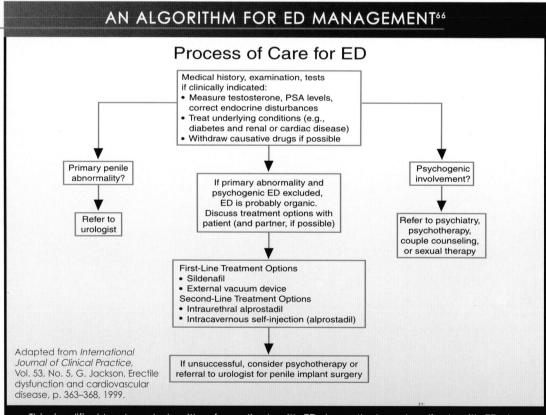

AN ALGORITHM FOR ED MANAGEMENT[66]

Process of Care for ED

Medical history, examination, tests if clinically indicated:
• Measure testosterone, PSA levels, correct endocrine disturbances
• Treat underlying conditions (e.g., diabetes and renal or cardiac disease)
• Withdraw causative drugs if possible

Primary penile abnormality?

Refer to urologist

If primary abnormality and psychogenic ED excluded, ED is probably organic. Discuss treatment options with patient (and partner, if possible)

Psychogenic involvement?

Refer to psychiatry, psychotherapy, couple counseling, or sexual therapy

First-Line Treatment Options
• Sildenafil
• External vacuum device
Second-Line Treatment Options
• Intraurethral alprostadil
• Intracavernous self-injection (alprostadil)

Adapted from *International Journal of Clinical Practice,* Vol. 53, No. 5, G. Jackson, Erectile dysfunction and cardiovascular disease, p. 363–368, 1999.

If unsuccessful, consider psychotherapy or referral to urologist for penile implant surgery

This simplified treatment algorithm for patients with ED shows that most patients with ED do not require sophisticated testing and can be effectively treated in the primary care setting.

Viagra enables erections following sexual stimulation and is given at dosages of 25, 50, or 100 mg taken as needed. The recommended starting dose for most patients is 50 mg. Patients need to be told that sexual stimulation is required for Viagra to work and that no more than 1 tablet should be taken within a 24-hour period.[6] The 100-mg dosage is preferred by many men to achieve maximal efficacy. If adverse side effects are noted with higher doses, then the 25-mg dose may be tried.[6] Onset of action occurs approximately 25 minutes following ingestion—longer if taken directly following a fatty meal.

When Viagra Should Never Be Used

Ever since Viagra was first approved, the labeling has warned that men who are also taking organic nitrates should never take the drug.[6] The reason: The two work via 2 different limbs of the same metabolic pathway, and the combination of the 2 drugs may lead to a sharp and potentially dangerous drop in blood pressure.[6]

Some Additional Cautions

Treatments for ED should not be used in men for whom sexual activity is inadvisable.

As noted previously, Viagra occasionally causes mild side effects, most of them related to the drug's vasodilating effects. The most common side effects are headache, flushing, and dyspepsia. Transient visual disturbances may infrequently occur.[6] There were rare postmarketing reports of priapism in men taking Viagra, often in combination with other ED therapies.

Furthermore, the labeling notes that men with certain conditions were excluded from the Viagra trials. Therefore, the drug should be prescribed with caution to men who have these conditions, which include retinitis pigmentosa, heart failure, heart disease causing unstable angina, extremes of blood pressure both high (>170/110) and low (<90/50), and recent experience (within the previous 6 months)

of an MI, stroke, or other life-threatening event.[6]

Drug-Drug Interaction

Viagra also can interact with certain drugs in addition to organic nitrates. Such interactions have been observed with co-administration of drugs that are metabolized by the same liver enzyme (cytochrome P450 isoform 3A4) that metabolizes Viagra. This can result in reduced clearance of Viagra and, hence, increased plasma levels of the drug. Drugs that can interact with Viagra in this way include erythromycin, cimetidine, ketoconazole, and the protease inhibitors, such as saquinavir and ritonavir. Viagra does not significantly affect the levels of these drugs, although Viagra blood levels may be affected. Concomitant use of ritonavir and Viagra can significantly increase blood levels of Viagra; the FDA-approved prescribing information for Viagra, updated in June 1999, recommends caution when prescribing Viagra to patients taking ritonavir. Such patients should not take more than 25 mg of Viagra in a 48-hour period.[6]

ED. Nevertheless, men with ED of unknown etiology still can be effectively treated.

The availability of Viagra has prompted a reevaluation of ED treatment methodology. Recognizing the need for evidence-based guidelines for managing patients with ED, a multidisciplinary panel of ED experts has examined the existing literature and practice standards. From this information, and by using the consensus process originally developed by the RAND Corporation, the panel developed a "process of care model for erectile dysfunction" to assist primary care physicians in choosing the most appropriate diagnostic tools and treatment interventions for optimizing the care of ED patients.[67] (Pfizer provided an independent educational grant for this work.)

The process of care model includes a stepwise decision-making approach to evaluating and treating patients with ED. Initial assessment

should include a careful clinical history, physical examination, and selected laboratory tests. The patient's treatment should be goal-oriented, taking into account the patient's and his partner's needs and preferences. With these criteria in mind, treatment should be tried in a stepwise fashion based on ease of administering the treatment, its reversibility, its relative invasiveness, and its cost.[67]

VIAGRA ACCEPTED AS FIRST-LINE TREATMENT FOR ED

One of Viagra's most impressive features is its effectiveness in treating ED whatever the cause, including ED due to diabetes, spinal cord injury, atherosclerosis, depression, and radical prostatectomy. This was a key reason why the process of care model recommended oral therapy, specifically Viagra, as a first-line treatment for ED.[67] Viagra has similarly been adopted as a first-line treatment for ED by the World Health Organization's First International

A TOUCH OF BLUE

Blue-tinged vision—the temporary side effect experienced by less than 3% of Viagra users[6]— has received considerable publicity. Less well known is that Pfizer scientists were well aware of this phenomenon and, long before Viagra was marketed, had conducted studies showing that this side effect was both transient and innocuous. (During clinical trials, increased sensitivity to light and blurred vision were reported, and they are listed as adverse events in the Viagra prescribing information.)

During the studies on sildenafil, doctors at Pfizer learned that the drug not only strongly inhibits the enzyme PDE 5, found mainly in the penis, but also has a weak (10-fold less) inhibitory effect on another PDE subtype: PDE 6, which is located exclusively in the retina[20,68] and plays a role in phototransduction. (See page 25 for a full list of phosphodiesterases.)

At this early stage, Pfizer doctors didn't know if the weak inhibition would produce visual symptoms. When clinical trials began, they realized that sildenafil was capable of "colorizing" vision.

"We noted this side effect early in the phase 1 clinical trials," says Dr. Peter Ellis, a senior project manager in the experimental medicine/early clinical group at Pfizer-Sandwich. "It was

consistently reported as a blue tinge to vision or as an increased perception of brightness, and it was clearly dose related."

The researchers didn't believe these visual effects would jeopardize sildenafil research, since they were consistently transient and reversible. Nevertheless, since the vision changes were related to sildenafil's mechanism of action, and since they involved the eye, "We knew it was vital that we carry out studies in more detail to define the consequences of these effects," said Dr. Ellis.

In these studies, volunteers were dosed with up to 200 mg of sildenafil— twice the maximum therapeutic dose and sufficient to produce visual symptoms in about 45% of subjects. The men were then given a wide range of visual function tests during the 1- to 4-hour period after taking the drug when visual symptoms are present.[68]

Color-vision testing revealed a dose-related and transient effect on subjects' ability to discriminate hues in the blue-green color range.[65] This was entirely consistent with the symptoms reported.

To assess possible permanent effects on vision, visual function testing was done on people enrolled in 2 long-term studies: before they took sildenafil and then after 12 weeks and again after 1 year of treatment. Subjects showed no change in any of the visual function tests over that time. In particular, there was no change from baseline in color-vision testing, clearly showing there was no long-term effect on color vision.[68]

This long-term testing also demonstrated that the visual effects were well tolerated. And while those patients reporting visual side effects would get them most times they took the drug, the effects were always transient and did not affect daily life.

Pfizer researchers also dosed animals with enough sildenafil to produce plasma levels some 65 times greater than levels present after giving 100 mg to patients, and they did so every day for a year.[65] This intense exposure had no effect on the animals' retinal tissue, which contains a similar enzyme to the PDE 6 found in human rods and cones.

"With this package of studies," says Dr. Ellis, "we are confident that sildenafil's visual effects are related to the inhibition of PDE 6, occur in a dose-related manner, are transient and reversible, and do not appear to represent a safety hazard."

Consultation on ED, the US Department of Veterans Affairs, and the Canadian Cardiovascular Society.

After Viagra had been on the market for only 18 months, it had already captured more than 90% of the market for ED treatments.[6] Who is taking Viagra? Market research shows that the overwhelming majority of those getting prescriptions for Viagra are men in the 40- to 70-year age group[6]—the people most likely to have a problem with ED and to benefit from using Viagra.

VIAGRA SPOTLIGHTS RELATIONSHIP BETWEEN SEX AND CARDIAC HEALTH

Viagra's postmarketing safety profile—following its use by more than 7 million men in the United States and 10 million around the world[6]—is generally consistent with the clinical trial data. That is also true for serious cardiovascular events such as myocardial infarction: As noted in Chapter 4, clinical trial results of double-blind studies showed no significant difference in the incidence of serious cardiovascular events between the

Viagra treatment groups and the control groups.[32] Nevertheless, anyone who has followed the press coverage of Viagra knows that the drug has been associated with deaths.[50]

Unfortunately, the press coverage of "Viagra deaths" rarely includes information that could put them into proper context:

- The FDA's adverse effects reporting system provides early warnings about problems associated with drugs but cannot determine the incidence of a problem. Reports to this voluntary system are uncontrolled and can come from sources such as friends, relatives, or neighbors of the patient—not just from doctors and pharmaceutical companies. Reports are also highly dependent on the publicity surrounding a novel drug.[47] Since Viagra experienced the most highly publicized drug launch in history, it is not surprising that the FDA received an unusually high number of reports.

- Most reports do not provide enough information to adequately assess causality. In many cases, all that is known is that a person at some time was prescribed Viagra; it is not known whether the prescription was filled, whether the person took Viagra, and, if he did take it, whether the dose occurred in close proximity to his death.

- By November 1998, about 6 million Viagra prescriptions had been written for 4.5 million men. At that time, the FDA Web site reported 130 deaths in men who had been prescribed Viagra.[48] Since high cholesterol, hypertension, and smoking are associated with both cardiovascular disease and ED, it is not suprising that men with ED are at risk for myocardial infarction—the cause of death for many of those reported to the FDA.

- Some of these deaths may be related to the concomitant—and strictly contraindicated—use of Viagra and organic nitrates.

- Perhaps most important, the majority of these men had preexisting cardiovascular risk factors. These risk factors, coupled with the added stress of sexual activity, are the most likely factors leading to these deaths. With more than 7000 man-years of experience in both double-blind and open-label trials, there is no evidence that Viagra increases the risk of myocardial infarction or death.[69]

KEEPING RISKS IN PERSPECTIVE

"Because men with cardiovascular disease are at increased risk of developing ED, and because ED and cardiovascular disease share important risk factors, attention has focused recently on the use of sildenafil in these men. . . .

"From the time of its approval in the United States in March 1998 through mid-November 1998, with approximately 6 million prescriptions written, 130 deaths were reported by the US Food and Drug Administration (FDA). Seventy-seven of the men who died had documented cardiovascular events. Sixteen men took or were administered nitroglycerin or an organic nitrate; 3 others had nitroglycerin in their possession. . . . A well-documented negative interaction between sildenafil and nitroglycerin and other organic nitrate compounds led to a clear statement of contraindication in the product's labeling. . . .

"Owing to this interaction . . . subjects were excluded from enrollment in the Phase II/III clinical trials of sildenafil if they were taking concomitant nitrate therapy. . . . The cardiovascular events (aside from flushing) reported in the placebo-controlled trials . . . were generally minor. . . . The incidence of serious cardiovascular events was also comparable between sildenafil- and placebo-treated patients. The rate of myocardial infarction was 1.7 per 100 person-years of treatment (95% CI, 0.8–2.6) in sildenafil-treated patients and 1.4 per 100 person-years of treatment (95% CI, 0.2–2.6) in placebo-treated patients. . . .

"Of the 130 men who died after receiving sildenafil, 90 had ≥ 1 risk factors for cardiovascular or cerebrovascular disease, including hypertension, hypercholesterolemia, diabetes mellitus, obesity, cigarette smoking, or a cardiac history. Three other patients without diagnosed heart disease or cardiovascular risk factors had evidence of severe coronary artery disease on autopsy. . . .

"It is difficult to draw firm conclusions from these data, given the lack of case controls, although given the high prevalence of cardiovascular disease in the United States, it does not appear that there was an excess of cardiovascular deaths in patients treated with sildenafil."

Excerpts from Kloner RA, Zusman RM. Cardiovascular effects of sildenafil citrate and recommendations for its use. Am J Cardiol. 1999;84:11N-17N.

ANNUAL RISK OF	ODDS
Dying from a plane falling on you	0.04 in 1 million[70]
Being killed by lightning	0.4 in 1 million[71]
Suffering a serious injury from your Christmas decorations	15.4 in 1 million[70]
Nonfatal MI within 2 hours of sexual activity*	100–200 in 1 million[72]
Dying in an auto accident	200 in 1 million[73]
Suffering a serious kitchen-knife injury	2000 in 1 million[70]
Serious injury from frequent use of exercise equipment	2500 in 1 million[70]
Being injured on stairs	3333 in 1 million[74]
Contracting a serious case of food poisoning	40,000 in 1 million[70]
Contracting a sexually transmitted disease	50,000 in 1 million[70]

*Based on the risk for a healthy man who engages in sexual activity once a week for a year, the odds (142 in 1 million) that a 50-year-old man will have a heart attack during the 2 hours following sex make that event somewhat less likely than dying in a traffic accident. The relative risk for men with and without prior heart disease is about the same, but the absolute risk can be increased by 5- to 10-fold.

EXERTION LEVEL OF SEXUAL ACTIVITY COMPARED WITH OTHER COMMON ACTIVITIES[72,75]

Estimated METs	Description	Physical Activities
2	Sitting	Reading, watching TV
3	Very light exertion	Moderate sexual activity with long-term partner, office work, strolling in park
4–5	Moderate exertion	Vigorous sexual activity, normal walking, golfing on foot, gardening, raking leaves
6–8	Vigorous to heavy exertion	Running, racquetball, fast biking, heavy snow-shoveling, competitive basketball

METs = metabolic equivalents of oxygen consumption

Sexual activity qualifies as moderate exertion.

Sexual activity slightly increases the risk for myocardial infarction, as shown by a recent epidemiologic study, which found that sexual intercourse increases a man's risk of an MI by a factor of about 2.5 (that is, a relative risk of 2.5) during the 2 hours following sex.[72] Among patients with a history of prior MI, the relative risk was 2.9, which was not significantly different from the risk among subjects without such a history.[72]

For a healthy 50-year-old man, this finding means that his "normal" 1-in-a-million risk of an MI during any 2-hour period rises to a 2.5-in-a-million risk in the 2-hour period following sex. Similarly, a man with a history of prior MI will see his customary 10-in-a-million risk of an MI increase to 29-in-a-million in the 2 hours after sex.[72]

Sexual activity in patients with preexisting heart disease may pose a potential cardiac risk. For some men, this risk is sufficiently high that they should avoid sexual activity.

The exertion required for sexual activity can range from 3 to 5 metabolic equivalents (METs), similar to that required for strolling in the park or normal walking (see chart above). Exercise treadmill testing may help to determine whether patients with coronary artery disease can achieve the workload associated with sexual intercourse.[69] Those men for whom sex is inadvisable should not be treated with ED therapy.

The good news is that most men can tolerate the physical stress of sexual activity. And men can further lower their already low risk of MI after sex by engaging in regular physical exercise.[72] Since exercise training lowers the peak heart rate during sex (or other moderate physical activity), it has a protective effect and may lower the potential for sexual activity to trigger MI.

TREATMENT OF ED: EFFECTS ON SEXUAL PARTNERS

When ED is successfully treated, the results may benefit not only the patient but also his sexual partner. This treatment may help couples recover the sexual intimacy in their relationships that may have been lost due to ED.

ED can cause depression, anxiety, and low self-esteem in men, and it can have a devastating effect on relationships as well. With the decline of sexual activity comes avoidance of other activities that help cement a relationship, including affectionate touching and other nonsexual types of communication.[76]

The man may blame his problem on his partner, who may in turn wonder if the man still loves her or may even suspect him of having an affair. The result may be mutual blame, a tacit agreement to avoid sex—and, ultimately, the end of the relationship.[76]

Ideally, treatment of sexual dysfunction should involve both partners in a relationship. Masters and Johnson made that point in their landmark 1970 text *Human Sexual Inadequacy*, in which they described sexual dysfunction as a couple's problem.[1] More recently, it has become clear that relationship problems not only may contribute to ED but can be a consequence of it.[76]

"Each couple presenting with ED has a unique history," says Dr. Sandra Leiblum, professor of clinical psychiatry and director of the Center for Sexual and Marital Health at the University of Medicine and Dentistry of New Jersey–Robert Wood Johnson Medical School in Piscataway, New Jersey. "It's important not to make assumptions regarding how important

PARTNER'S PERSPECTIVE

The priceless benefit of restored sexual function is explained beautifully by the wife of one man treated with Viagra:

Robert and Judy Leslie of Garden Grove, California, have been married for 36 years. For nearly 23 of those years, Robert has been confined to a wheelchair due to an accident that left him paraplegic.

"Going for a walk, holding hands, a walk on the beach, those are all gone. Plus your physical, your sexual life: It's not gone, but it's a new life that you have to learn to live with. He used to come up behind me and put his arm around me and kiss me on my neck. Little things that people take for granted," says Judy, who goes on to describe a most memorable visit to her family physician last year.

JUDY AND ROBERT LESLIE
"The first night we used Viagra, we both ended up crying because it was so special. . . ."

"I was in the office and the doctor called me in to one of the rooms and he said that a new product had come out. He explained to me what it was and said, 'I want you to take it and try it.' And I said, 'But there's been nothing for 22½ years.' He said, 'Just take it and try it.'

"So we decided Friday was date night. We had a nice dinner and took the phone off the hook, and he took the Viagra and it worked beautifully. After 22½ years of not being able to have physical relations, it was just like a honeymoon. I have to be honest. The first night we used it, we both ended up crying because it was so special and it was beautiful and we knew each other so well but yet we were both very nervous because we didn't know what to expect. And after that many years of not having what you would really call an intimate moment, it was beautiful to be able to make love to your husband and feel like a woman again. It was very exciting.

"When we go to bed now, whether we use Viagra or not, there is still a lot of laughter, a lot of playing. There's a lot more than there ever was before. And that's what's fun."

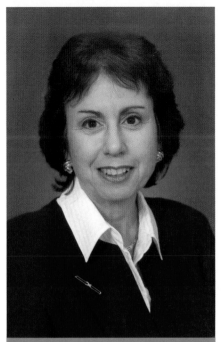

SANDRA LEIBLUM, PhD
Professor of Clinical Psychiatry and Director of the Center for Sexual and Marital Health, University of Medicine and Dentistry of New Jersey–Robert Wood Johnson Medical School

sexual intercourse is to the individuals in the relationship affected by ED.

"For some couples, sex is extremely important; for others, the importance of sex is minimal. You need to know the situation before making treatment recommendations. For example, you would certainly want to recommend ED treatment for couples for whom sex cements the quality of their relationship.

"It's also important to ask how long there has been a lack of sexual activity and what the reasons are for that lack. If a couple hasn't had sexual contact because of anger and dissension in the relationship, then you may want to see resolution of those issues before addressing ED treatment.

"When a couple has not had sexual intercourse for a long time, they need to start back gradually. That's why, when integrating treatment with Viagra into a relationship, you need to help the couple create an atmosphere in which intercourse is not considered the main event but rather as something that can occur if all the preceding steps have been carried out in a comfortable manner."

Viagra is not a magic potion for restoring relationships. It does not increase sexual desire and will not work without sexual stimulation. But by restoring a man's erectile function, Viagra can restore the sexual component that may be a crucial part of a couple's overall relationship. ●

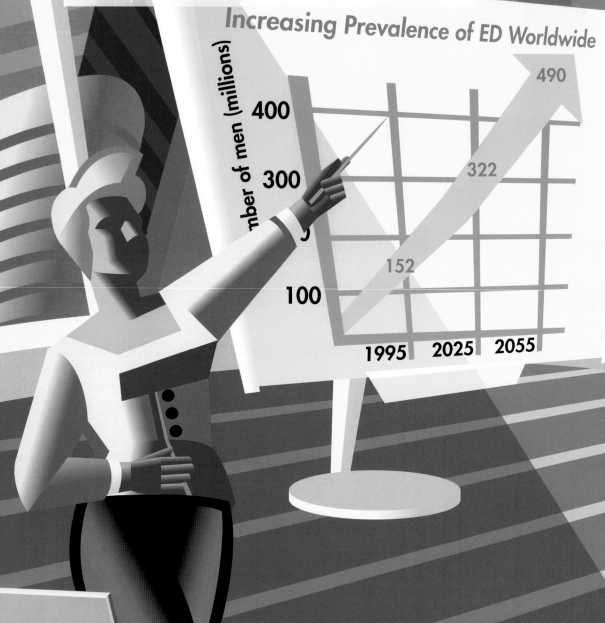

A medical school classroom of the future. The professor says, "It's hard to believe, but sexual health has been part of the standard medical education and medical history only since about 2001, shortly after the arrival of Viagra (sildenafil citrate). Looking at the increasing prevalence of erectile dysfunction in recent decades, it's more critical than ever that we take the time to take a sexual history."

Increasing Prevalence of ED Worldwide

Number of men (millions)

400

300

100

490

322

152

1995 2025 2055

FACTOID: By 2025, the worldwide total of men experiencing erectile dysfunction will have more than doubled, from an estimated 152 million in 1995 to a projected 322 million.[77]

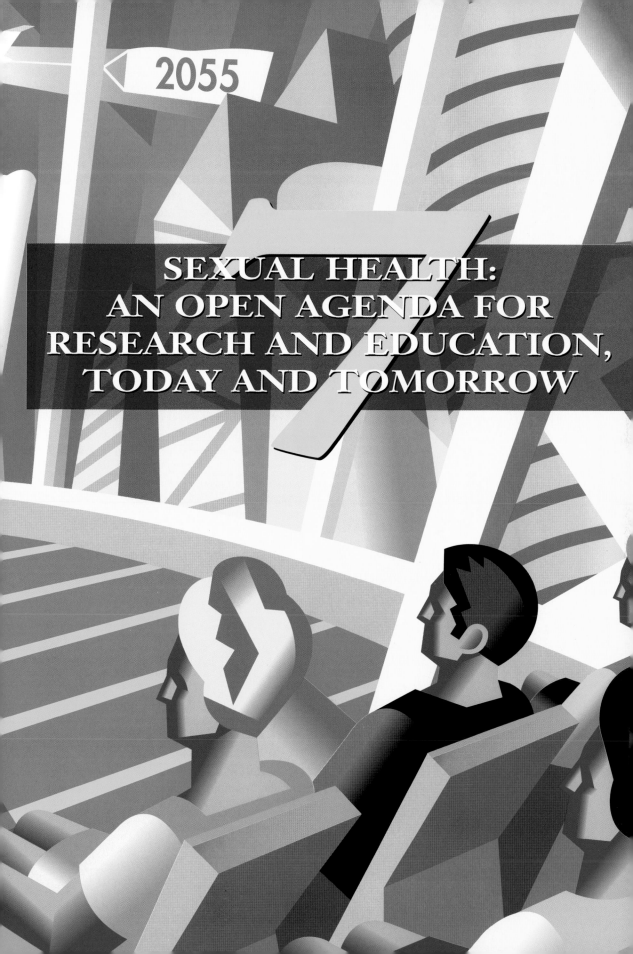

2055

SEXUAL HEALTH:
AN OPEN AGENDA FOR
RESEARCH AND EDUCATION,
TODAY AND TOMORROW

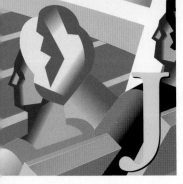

Just as sexual function has been a taboo topic in society as a whole, the medical profession also has largely avoided dealing with it. Before Viagra (sildenafil citrate), erectile dysfunction (ED) was generally the province of those few urologists and mental health professionals who specialized in treating sexual dysfunction. Viagra has taken this rather esoteric field and broadened it tremendously. Today, doctors diagnosing and treating ED include not only the aforementioned specialists but also many others, including primary care physicians, internists, cardiologists, endocrinologists, and geriatricians.

Medicine's renewed focus on ED has already resulted in some major practical benefits for patients:

- *ED can signal a serious medical condition.* By drawing millions of men with ED into doctors' offices, Viagra has presented both doctor and patient with a potentially lifesaving opportunity to see whether a man's ED could be a symptom of an undiagnosed but potentially serious underlying condition, such as atherosclerosis or diabetes.[2,62,78]

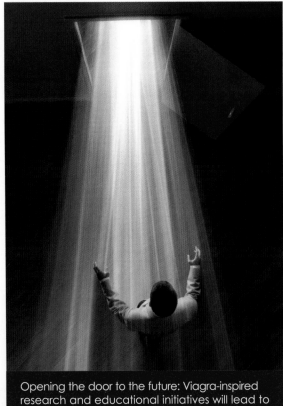

Opening the door to the future: Viagra-inspired research and educational initiatives will lead to a better understanding of sexual health.

- *Help is available.* Before Viagra, many men with ED were unaware that anything could be done. They now know that ED is a treatable condition.

- *Sex can be risky.* The media attention on Viagra has highlighted the fact that sex is a moderately strenuous activity that can increase the risk of myocardial infarction (MI)—especially in someone with underlying heart disease or a history of MI.[72] While the absolute risk of MI following sexual activity is very low,[72] coronary artery disease itself is common.[79] A conversation should take place between patients with heart disease and their doctors about whether the man can safely engage in sexual activity. Thanks to the new focus on sexual health, that crucial conversation may now be happening more often.

BEYOND PATIENT CARE

The new focus on sexual health engendered by Viagra has greatly stimulated research interest in ED as well. Previously, scientists who studied sexual physiology could expect to receive little respect from their colleagues and virtually nothing in the way of federal funding. With the advent of Viagra, research interest in sexual functioning in general and ED in particular has soared.[80]

Already, these research efforts are yielding a better understanding of erectile physiology and the underlying causes of ED—plus intensified efforts among pharmaceutical companies to develop products to compete with Viagra. The main beneficiaries of all this research will be patients with ED and their partners.

As effective as Viagra is, research into possible additional health benefits and treatment indications is far from over. "For every compound we develop and market, we try to increase its value to patients, physicians, and to us," says Dr. Pierre Wicker, US team leader for Viagra clinical trials, Pfizer Central Research, Groton, Connecticut. "We keep conducting studies to improve our understanding of a compound's efficacy and safety and to find new indications and new uses."

Some of these Viagra studies are part of the phase 4 clinical work that typically begins once any drug is approved. The studies done early in phase 4 usually compare the recently approved drug with similar drugs that treat the same problem. But with Viagra, that has not been easy to do.

"One of the many unique things about Viagra is that it's the first in its class—the first oral medication for treating ED," says Dr. Richard Siegel, medical director at Pfizer headquarters in New York City. "We don't really have a competitor against which we can compare Viagra, so it has been a challenge to come up with studies of this kind."

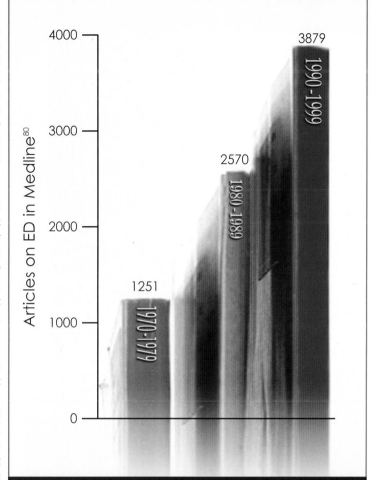

MEDICAL LITERATURE REFLECTS INCREASED INTEREST IN ED

Articles on ED in Medline[80]

- 1970-1979: 1251
- 1980-1989: 2570
- 1990-1999: 3879

The number of medical articles published on ED has been increasing and should continue to grow with ongoing Viagra-inspired research.

Pfizer has proceeded with other types of trials commonly done following a drug's approval. Some of these studies focus on special groups, such as racial or ethnic minorities. Other studies may result in new treatment indications for Viagra.

VIAGRA IN VARIOUS ETHNIC GROUPS

Pfizer recently completed a clinical trial involving African-American men with ED. Also in late 1999, Pfizer implemented a clinical study involving Hispanic-American men with ED. These 2 studies are expected to confirm Viagra's efficacy, as already demonstrated by clinical trials conducted worldwide.

HELP FOR PROSTATE CANCER PATIENTS

In the clinical studies leading to Viagra's approval, men with ED after radical prostatectomy saw improved erections with the medication. However, Viagra efficacy rates in these men were not as high as for men with ED due to other etiologies (43% efficacy in radical prostatectomy vs. 83% efficacy in spinal cord injury, for example).[6] In 2000, a new study was reported, which focused more carefully on the type of surgery performed and respective efficacy of Viagra. It was found that "the use of sildenafil offers a

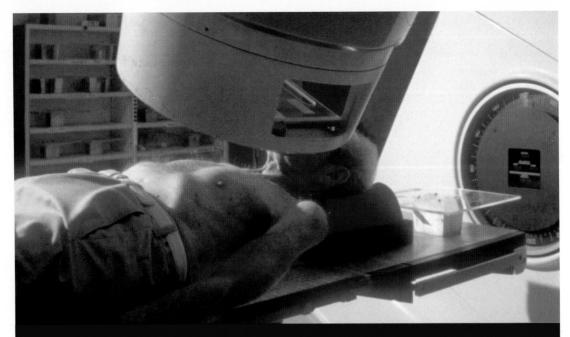

Several studies have demonstrated Viagra's usefulness in men who have ED due to radiation treatment for prostate cancer.

chance to salvage roughly 70% of our impotent, motivated patients if a bilateral [nerve-sparing] procedure is done." Furthermore, unilateral nerve-sparing procedures allowed 50% of patients to benefit from Viagra.[81]

Recently published post–FDA approval studies indicate that Viagra works not only for post–radical prostatectomy patients but also for prostate cancer patients who have undergone radiation therapy, as indicated in the table below.

CAN INJECTION-THERAPY PATIENTS BE SWITCHED TO VIAGRA?

Before Viagra became available, intracavernosal self-injection therapy was considered the state-of-the-art treatment for ED. After Viagra's approval, some physicians wondered if patients taking injection therapy could be successfully switched to the oral medication. A recent study compared Viagra's effectiveness in men who had previously been treated with injection therapy and men who had not. Both groups of men experienced significant—and similar—improvements in erectile function with Viagra.[86]

Another clinical study, which included 42 men who were satisfied with self-injection therapy and 87 men who were not, found that similar percentages of both groups (62% and 56%, respectively) were satisfied with Viagra.[87]

Viagra may also be the answer for some men who have not been helped by self-injection

OPEN-LABEL STUDIES OF VIAGRA FOR MEN WITH ED DUE TO RADIATION TREATMENT OF PROSTATE CANCER

TYPE OF INTERVENTION	NUMBER OF SUBJECTS	% IMPROVEMENT IN ERECTILE FUNCTION WITH VIAGRA
External beam radiotherapy[82]	35	77
External beam radiotherapy[83]	50	74
Brachytherapy (radioactive seed implantation)[84]	62	81
External beam radiotherapy or brachytherapy[85]	21	71

VIAGRA AND MALE REPRODUCTION

While ED prevalence increases with age, the condition is certainly not limited to men over 40. Particularly in younger men, a devastating consequence of ED may be the inability to father a child. Now, men with ED due to type 1 diabetes, spinal cord injury, depression, and other causes may have the capacity to have successful intercourse using Viagra.

Recently, 2 small studies indicated that Viagra was valuable for men participating in assisted-reproduction techniques (such as intrauterine insemination and in vitro fertilization).[89,90] "In these cases," the authors wrote, "the use of Viagra was planned in advance and it successfully solved any unpredictable erectile dysfunction on the day of insemination."[89] In another study, a single 100-mg dose of Viagra had no effect on sperm motility or morphology.[6]

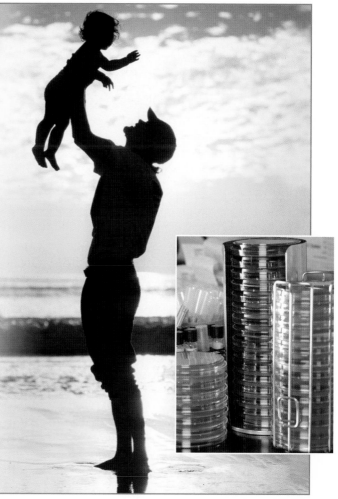

therapy. A study of 93 such men found that 32 of them (34% of the group) responded to Viagra.[88]

EXPLORING THE RELATIONSHIPS AMONG ED, DEPRESSION, AND VIAGRA USE

ED and depression often occur together, and the relationship between these conditions is complex and bidirectional. Studies have shown that men with ED are at increased risk for depression.[91,92] In fact, ED, lack of sexual desire, and decreased sexual activity are considered symptoms of depression.[93,94]

A recently completed placebo-controlled study demonstrated that Viagra is effective and well tolerated in men suffering from both ED and depression.[95,96] Interestingly, men who responded to ED

treatment in this study—whether they were taking Viagra or placebo—experienced significant reductions of depressive symptoms as measured by the Hamilton Depression Rating Scale.[91]

EFFECT OF ALLEVIATION OF ED ON DEPRESSIVE SYMPTOMS AT 12 WEEKS[95]

	Baseline	ED Optimal Responder (n=58)	ED Nonresponder (n=78)
HAM-D	16.7	6.4*	14.2
BDI	15.6	6.4*	13.7

*$P<0.0001$ vs ED nonresponders (ANOVA)

Men who responded to ED treatment, whether they took Viagra or placebo, experienced significant reductions of depressive symptoms as measured by 2 validated scales.

In addition, Viagra may prove helpful in alleviating the ED that is often a side effect when men take antidepressant medications. Several small open-label studies have shown that men with antidepressant-associated ED experienced significant improvements in erectile function after taking Viagra.[97,98]

ED AND RENAL DIALYSIS PATIENTS: EXPLORING THE CONNECTION

"It's generally assumed that patients with renal disease of any type have difficulty with sexual function, but there is really no good study to show that," says Dr. Eric Grossman, medical director at Pfizer and a board-certified nephrologist. Epidemiologists at the University of Pennsylvania have conducted a study to examine the prevalence of ED among dialysis patients. "This study may also help us begin to understand whether the ED in these patients results from their renal failure per se, or from the cause of their kidney failure, or other factors," Dr. Grossman says.

In research now in progress, Pfizer is studying the pharmacokinetics of Viagra in hemodialysis patients. Once those data are in hand, the company hopes to launch placebo-controlled

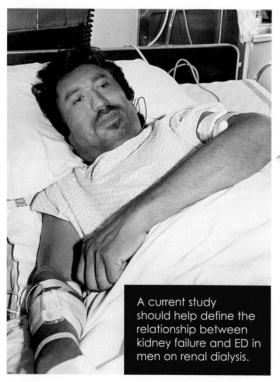

A current study should help define the relationship between kidney failure and ED in men on renal dialysis.

clinical trials in which Viagra will be tested in dialysis patients.

MATTERS OF THE HEART

Two interesting studies related to Viagra were recently reported. The first study evaluated the effect of a single dose of Viagra on the blood vessels of patients with moderate heart failure. Compared with placebo, patients receiving 12.5 mg of Viagra experienced slight improvement in endothelial function within the brachial artery, while patients receiving 25 mg or 50 mg of Viagra had more noticeable improvement. Those with impaired endothelial function include patients with atherosclerosis, diabetes, and hypertension. The clinical significance of these findings is not clear but, at the very least, they indicate that Viagra does not adversely affect endothelial function.[99]

The second study, conducted in animals at the University of Minnesota, showed that Viagra use increased coronary blood flow with no change in distal coronary pressure after applying coronary stenosis. The authors suggest that these findings indicate that Viagra should be well tolerated in patients with underlying coronary artery disease, but the clinical significance of the findings remains to be shown.[100]

FUTURE RESEARCH DIRECTIONS IN UNDERSTANDING AND TREATING SEXUAL DYSFUNCTION

The advent of an effective oral treatment for male sexual dysfunction has also raised broader questions that researchers will try to answer in the coming years: Can ED be prevented by medical intervention? Is there a safe and effective medical treatment for female sexual dysfunction?

While investigators at universities and pharmaceutical companies press forward to answer these questions, social scientists, educators, and medical economists are posing additional relevant questions: How important is sexual functioning to an individual, a relationship, and society? Should health insurance companies reimburse the cost of treating sexual dysfunction? How can educational initiatives about sexual dysfunction be more effective?

SPREADING THE WORD ABOUT ED: AN EMPHASIS ON EDUCATION

Research into sexual health is only an academic exercise unless physicians and the public learn and incorporate into practice what is already known about sexual dysfunction and its treatment. To that end, the ongoing Viagra research program is taking place in tandem with efforts to educate both physicians and the public about sexual health.

Pfizer has made a major investment in educating physicians about this topic, starting with the training they receive in medical school. "We would like to help medical schools improve the way medical students are educated about both male and female sexual dysfunction, since whatever time is spent on sexual health is usually limited to sexually transmitted diseases or reproductive matters," says Dr. Grossman. "We have contacted 15 of the top medical schools in the country and found that more than half of them expressed positive interest in developing a sexual health/sexual dysfunction curriculum." As a result, Pfizer is planning to provide funding for medical schools to develop such curricula.

"As a leader in sexual health, it is our responsibility at Pfizer to make sure that the information we and the academic leaders in the field have is fully available to physicians in the US and throughout the world," says Dr. Grossman.

Independent continuing medical education (CME) programs have been initiated aimed at educating physicians and other healthcare professionals about sexual health. Examples of these educational efforts include CME symposia at annual meetings

SEXUAL EDUCATION IN MEDICAL SCHOOL: THEN, NOW, AND TOMORROW

"There was a tremendous push in the early 1970s to include sexual education in the medical schools," says Dr. Gerald Melchiode, author of *Beyond Viagra* and a clinical professor of psychiatry at the University of Texas Southwestern Medical Center in Dallas. He remembers taking part in one such teaching effort at Hahnemann Medical College in Philadelphia.

"I was involved in teaching a 36-hour course on human sexuality for second-year students," he says.

"It was an amazing course, which I taught with urologists and gynecologists. We discussed sexual adjustment following medical illnesses and after surgery and had panels on sex and religion. I also taught human sexuality to house staff, so I worked with urology residents, ob-gyn residents, and family practice residents. We sat down with them, watched them do interviews, and helped them in counseling patients. Such programs started to become part of the curriculum of medical education. Subsequently, however, they have all been dismantled.

"Today," says Dr. Melchiode, "there are occasional lectures, but they're embedded in other courses. For example, you might have a lecture on the human sexual response in the physiology course or the endocrine course. Or there might be a lecture on taking a sexual history in the human behavior course. But they don't all come together for the student, and there is nowhere in medical education where somebody goes over how to take a sexual history with a medical student."

Despite this negative observation, Dr. Melchiode is encouraged by the spotlight Viagra has

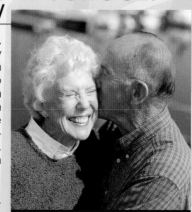

Comprehensive sexual education programs in medical schools will likely teach physicians that no one is "too old for sex."

placed on sexual health education. "With comprehensive new medical school programs, physicians may become much more knowledgeable about sexuality and sexual problems than they are now, and no longer tell patients they are 'too old to worry about sex' and will understand that nobody is too old. Couples could routinely continue to have regular sexual intercourse into their 80s and 90s."

of professional organizations, direct-mail CME monographs to primary care physicians nationwide, and national audioconferences that allow physicians to call in to listen to a lecture about ED and ask questions of an expert.

FROM PROFESSIONAL TO PUBLIC EDUCATION

While physicians themselves are becoming educated about sexual health, they also need to be able to teach their patients about the subject. To make this an easier task, Pfizer has developed lecture programs and written materials to help physicians educate their patients about ED. Brochures, slide kits, and anatomic diagrams and models can help physicians explain to patients that ED is a medical condition that can be treated. Still, many people either do not understand the problem or feel too strong a stigma to seek treatment for it.

"Millions of men with ED have had the courage to step forward and get treated with Viagra," says Dr. Mike Sweeney, medical director at Pfizer. "But we also know there are huge numbers of men out there who are bothered by ED but have not yet sought treatment.

"Up until now, men who have been treated with Viagra are typically older men who have had ED for a longer time," says Dr. Sweeney. "The much larger group of men with untreated ED are relatively younger and relatively healthier men aged 40 through 60. For them, their moderate or mild ED is not so severe a disability that they're willing to overcome the social stigma they associate with impotence and to seek help for their problem.

"We want to reach these men—through advertisements, pamphlets, lectures—and educate them about ED so they'll feel more comfortable about going to their doctor, getting diagnosed, getting treated—and getting a new lease on life," stresses Dr. Sweeney.

A REMARKABLE TALE OF SCIENCE AND SERENDIPITY

The story of Viagra epitomizes modern pharmaceutical research at its best. Viagra was first of all the fruit of rational drug design: Pfizer researchers wanted a drug that would inhibit the enzyme phosphodiesterase type 5 (PDE 5), since it was known that blocking this enzyme resulted in actions that theoretically would have beneficial cardiac effects, including decreased vascular resistance and reduced platelet aggregation. After synthesizing nearly 1500 chemicals, the researchers decided that an entity they dubbed sildenafil citrate was the best candidate for the job.

Then came clinical studies in which sildenafil was tested on healthy volunteers and angina patients and produced mild hemodynamic effects—reduced systolic and diastolic blood pressure without clinically significant changes in cardiac output.

Sildenafil seemed fated to gather dust on a laboratory shelf. But in a dramatic proof of the axiom that "fortune favors the prepared mind," it was saved by an observation: Some of the healthy volunteers in phase 1 studies experienced erections after taking the drug.

And so began sildenafil's journey from experimental angina drug to the world's first pill for ED. That effort required the participation of hundreds of Pfizer employees, 192 investigators at prominent medical institutions worldwide, and nearly 4500 patients enrolled in 21 clinical trials in 13 countries. As noted in this chapter, that research effort is continuing, so the journey is far from over.

Viagra, the culmination of all this effort, has been a very successful drug. The drug's true measure of success can be seen in the millions of men who have regained the ability to have erections and the millions of relationships that have benefited as a result.

A TABLET THAT TRANSFORMS LIVES

Only the early returns are in, but the trend is abundantly clear. By restoring erectile function to millions of men, Viagra has had a tremendous impact on people's lives. Thanks in no small part to Viagra itself, the truth about ED has finally been recognized: This widespread problem can cause tremendous anguish.

ED can severely damage a man's self-esteem—even his very identity. It can cause depression and anxiety, bitterness and withdrawal. With Viagra, men who had resigned themselves to "impotence" have now recovered a part of living they may have believed to be gone forever.

A Tablet That Has Transformed Sex in Society

It's truly mind-boggling when you think about it: A former United States senator and presidential candidate appeared on CNN's *Larry King Live* to tell the nation about his ED and its successful treatment with Viagra. And who could have predicted that ED would come up constantly in late-night television monologues, be featured as a cover story in magazines, and even function as a subplot on TV dramas?

ED has long been a topic so fraught with shame that it went unmentioned even in bedrooms and doctors' offices. Now, almost overnight, Viagra has legitimized ED, transforming it from a private agony to a very public medical problem.

Raising the public's consciousness about ED surely ranks as one of Viagra's major contributions. But even more important is Viagra's impact on the lives of some 7 million men in the United States, and 10 million around the world, who have been able to deal with their ED by taking a pill.[6] So it's not surprising that *USA Today*, in an article commemorating Viagra's first year on the market, called it "the little blue tablet that has triggered a sexual revolution" and predicted that "life in the USA, and in more than 50 other countries in which it's marketed, will never be the same."[101]

"Sexual revolution" might be too strong a term if Viagra's influence were limited to publicizing ED and successfully treating men with the problem. But as the *USA Today* article noted, Viagra has done even more than that, and its impact on society will continue for a long time to come.[101]

"I think Viagra has been an extraordinary social phenomenon," says John Bancroft, director of the Kinsey Institute for Research in Sex, Gender, and Reproduction in Bloomington, Indiana. "It has opened up discussion about ordinary sexual function. It has raised this whole question about the relevance of sex to middle years and later years and its priority in relation to healthcare and insurance coverage. Just in terms of how we think about male sexuality, it's had an impact that's still resounding."[101] ●

REFERENCES

1. Masters W, Johnson V. *Human Sexual Inadequacy*. Boston, MA: Little, Brown and Company; 1970: 137–160.

2. DeWire DM. Evaluation and treatment of erectile dysfunction. *Am Fam Physician*. 1996;53:2101–2108.

3. NIH Consensus Development Panel on Impotence. Impotence. *JAMA*. 1993;270:83–90.

4. World Health Organization. *Education and Treatment in Human Sexuality: The Training of Health Professionals*. Geneva, Switzerland: World Health Organization; 1975. Technical Report Series, No. 572.

5. Feldman HA, Goldstein I, Hatzichristou DG, Krane RJ, McKinlay JB. Impotence and its medical and psychosocial correlates: results of the Massachusetts male aging study. *J Urol*. 1994;151:54–61.

6. Data on file, Pfizer Inc., New York, NY.

7. Brindley GS. Cavernosal alpha-blockade: a new technique for investigating and treating erectile impotence. *Br J Psychiatry*. 1983;143:332–337.

8. Sundaram CP, Thomas W, Pryor LE, Sidi AA, Billups K, Pryor JL. Long-term follow-up of patients receiving injection therapy for erectile dysfunction. *Urology*. 1997;49:932–935.

9. Flynn RJ, Williams G. Long-term follow-up of patients with erectile dysfunction commenced on self injection with intracavernosal papaverine with or without phentolamine. *Br J Urol*. 1996;78:628–631.

10. Weiss JN, Badlani GH, Ravalli R, Brettschneider N. Reasons for high drop-out rate with self-injection therapy for impotence. *Int J Impot Res*. 1994;6: 171–174.

11. Jackson G, Benjamin N, Jackson N, Allen MJ. Effects of sildenafil citrate on human hemodynamics. *Am J Cardiol*. 1999;83:13C–20C.

12. Terrett NK, Bell AS, Brown D, Ellis P. Sildenafil (Viagra™), a potent and selective inhibitor of type 5 cGMP phosphodiesterase with utility for the treatment of male erectile dysfunction. *Biorg Med Chem Let*. 1996;6:1819–1824.

13. Ignarro LJ, Bush PA, Buga GM, Wood KS, Fukuto JM, Rajfer J. Nitric oxide and cyclic GMP formation upon electrical field stimulation cause relaxation of corpus cavernosum smooth muscle. *Biochem Biophys Res Commun*. 1990;170:843–850.

14. Bush PA, Aronson WJ, Buga GM, Rajfer J, Ignarro LJ. Nitric oxide is a potent relaxant of human and rabbit corpus cavernosum. *J Urol*. 1992;147:1650–1655.

15. Webb DJ, Freestone S, Allen MJ, Muirhead GJ. Sildenafil citrate and blood-pressure-lowering drugs: results of drug interaction studies with an organic nitrate and a calcium antagonist. *Am J Cardiol*. 1999;83:21C–28C.

16. Rajfer J, Aronson WJ, Bush PA, Dorey FJ, Ignarro LJ. Nitric oxide as a mediator of relaxation of the corpus cavernosum in response to nonadrenergic, noncholinergic neurotransmission. *N Engl J Med*. 1992;326:90–94.

17. Levine LA, Lenting EL. Use of nocturnal penile tumescence and rigidity in the evaluation of male erectile dysfunction. *Urol Clin North Am*. 1995;22: 775–788.

18. Boolell M, Gepi-Attee S, Gingell JC, Allen MJ. Sildenafil, a novel effective oral therapy for male erectile dysfunction. *Br J Urol*. 1996;78:257–261.

19. Rulten SL, Dapling A, Lanfear J, et al. Isolation of a human phosphodiesterase 5 CDNA and in situ analysis of its expression in human corpus cavernosum. *J Urol*. 1998;159(suppl):92.

20. Wallis RM, Corbin JD, Francis SH, Ellis P. Tissue distribution of phosphodiesterase families and the effects of sildenafil on tissue cyclic nucleotides, platelet function, and the contractile responses of trabeculae carneae and aortic rings in vitro. *Am J Cardiol*. 1999;83:3C–12C.

21. Burnett AL. Nitric oxide in the penis: physiology and pathology. *J Urol*. 1997;157:320–324.

22. Rosen RC, Riley A, Wagner G, Osterloh IH, Kirkpatrick, J, Mishra A. The International Index of Erectile Function (IIEF): a multidimensional scale for assessment of erectile dysfunction. *Urology*. 1997;49:822–830.

23. Gingell C, Jardin A, Olsson AM, et al, and the Multicentre Study Group. A new oral treatment for erectile dysfunction: a double-blind, placebo-controlled, once daily dose response study [abstract]. *Proc Am Urol Assoc*. 1996;155(suppl):495A. Abstract 738.

24. Christiansen E, and the Multicentre Study Group; Hodges M, Hollingshead M, Kirkpatrick J, Dickinson S, Osterloh I. Sildenafil (Viagra™) a new oral treatment for erectile dysfunction (ED): results of a 16 week open dose escalation study [abstract]. *Int J Impot Res*. 1996;8(3):147.

25. Young S, for the Sildenafil Study Group. Partner's perceptions of the efficacy of sildenafil (Viagra) in the treatment of erectile dysfunction. Poster presented at: 28th British Congress of Obstetrics and Gynaecology; June 30–July 3, 1998; Harrogate, United Kingdom.

26. Maytom M, Orr M, Osterloh I, et al. Sildenafil (Viagra)—an oral treatment for men with erectile dysfunction caused by traumatic spinal cord injury: a two-stage, double-blind, placebo-controlled study to assess the efficacy and safety of sildenafil [abstract]. *Br J Urol*. 1997;80(2):94.

27. Derry F, Gardner BP, Glass C, et al. Sildenafil (Viagra): a double-blind, placebo-controlled, single-dose, two-way crossover study in men with erectile dysfunction caused by traumatic spinal cord injury. *J Urol*. 1997;157(suppl):181.

28. Price DE, Gingell JC, Gepi-Attee S, et al. Sildenafil: study of a novel oral treatment for erectile dysfunction in diabetic men. *Diabet Med*. 1998;15(10):821–825.

29. Feldman R, and the Sildenafil Study Group. Sildenafil in the treatment of erectile dysfunction: efficacy in patients taking concomitant antihypertensive therapy. *Am J Hypertens*. 1998;11(4 pt 2).

30. Morales A, Gingell C, Collins M, Wicker PA, Osterloh IH. Clinical safety of oral sildenafil citrate (Viagra) in the treatment of erectile dysfunction. *Int J Impot Res*. 1998;10:69–74.

31. Rendell MS, Rajfer J, Wicker PA, Smith MD, for the Sildenafil Diabetes Study Group. Sildenafil for treatment of erectile dysfunction in men with diabetes. *JAMA*. 1999;281:421–426.

32. Zusman RM, Morales A, Glasser DB, Osterloh IH. Overall cardiovascular profile of sildenafil citrate. *Am J Cardiol*. 1999;83(5A):35C–44C.

33. Padma-Nathan H, Steers WD, Wicker PA, for the

Sildenafil Study Group. Efficacy and safety of oral sildenafil in the treatment of erectile dysfunction: a double-blind, placebo-controlled study of 329 patients. *Int J Clin Pract*. 1998;52:375–380.

34. Utiger RD. A pill for impotence. *N Engl J Med*. 1998;338:1458–1459.

35. Conti CR, Pepine CJ, Sweeney M. Efficacy and safety of sildenafil citrate in the treatment of erectile dysfunction in patients with ischemic heart disease. *Am J Cardiol*. 1999;83:29C–34C.

36. Derry FA, Dinsmore WW, Fraser M, et al. Efficacy and safety of oral sildenafil (Viagra) in men with erectile dysfunction caused by spinal cord injury. *Neurology*. 1998;51:1629–1633.

37. Zippe CD, Kedia AW, Kedia K, Nelson DR, Agarwal A. Treatment of erectile dysfunction after radical prostatectomy with sildenafil citrate (Viagra). *Urology*. 1998;52:963–966.

38. Price D, for the Sildenafil Study Group. Sildenafil citrate (Viagra) efficacy in the treatment of erectile dysfunction in patients with common concomitant conditions. *Int J Clin Pract*. 1999;102(suppl):21–23.

39. Shabsigh R, for the Sildenafil Study Group. Efficacy of sildenafil (Viagra) is not affected by etiology of erectile dysfunction. *Int J Impot Res*. 1998;10(suppl 3):S32.

40. Goldstein I, Lue TF, Padma-Nathan H, Rosen RC, Steers WD, Wicker PA, for the Sildenafil Study Group. Oral sildenafil in the treatment of erectile dysfunction. *N Engl J Med*. 1998;338:1397–1404.

41. Auerbach S, for the Sildenafil and Multicentre Study Groups. Sildenafil (Viagra) in the treatment of erectile dysfunction: efficacy in elderly patients. Poster presented at: American Geriatrics Society Annual Scientific Meeting; May 1998; Seattle, WA.

42. Giuliano F, Jardin A, Gingell CJ, et al, and the Multicentre Study Group. Sildenafil (Viagra), an oral treatment for erectile dysfunction: a 1-year, open-label extension study. *Br J Urol*. 1997;80:93.

43. Hackett G, Gingell C, and the Multicentre Study Group. Long-term safety and efficacy after 2 years of Viagra (sildenafil citrate) treatment in erectile dysfunction and the overall incidence of myocardial infarction. Poster presented at: American Urological Association 93rd Annual Meeting, May 30–June 4, 1998; San Diego, CA.

44. Food and Drug Administration. *FDA Approves Impotence Pill, Viagra*. Rockville, MD: National Press Office; March 27, 1998. Talk Paper T98-14.

45. Food and Drug Administration. *FDA Drug Approvals in 1997 Set New Records*. Rockville, MD: National Press Office; January 14, 1998. Talk Paper T98-2.

46. Beard S. 'Capitalize' Social Security to create a nation of shareholders. *The Baltimore Sun*. March 11, 1996; Editorial:7A.

47. Food and Drug Administration. *The Clinical Impact of Adverse Event Reporting*. Rockville, MD: Center for Drug Evaluation and Research; October 1996. A MedWatch Continuing Education Article.

48. Food and Drug Administration Web site. Post-marketing safety of sildenafil citrate (Viagra). Available at: http://www.fda.gov/cder/consumerinfo/viagra/safety3.htm. Accessed December 3, 1999.

49. Weber J, Barrett A, Mandel M, Laderman J. The new era of lifestyle drugs. *Business Week*. May 11, 1998:92–98.

50. Lore D. Overcoming impotence. *Atlanta Journal and Constitution*. May 17, 1998:6C.

51. *Montreal Gazette* [editorial]. Cited in: Viagra fever: much is in your mind. *USA Today*. May 1, 1998.

52. Viagra: on release. *BMJ*. 1998;317:759–760.

53. Butler RN. The Viagra revolution. *Geriatrics*. 1998;53(10):8–9.

54. Laumann EO, Paik A, Rosen RC. Sexual dysfunction in the United States. *JAMA*. 1999;281:537–544.

55. New survey finds nearly four and one half million men experienced sexual dysfunction [press release]. Emmaus, PA: National Men's Health Week; June 14, 1999.

56. Jacoby S. Great sex: what's age got to do with it? AARP Web site. Available at: http://www.aarp.org/mmaturity/sept_oct99/greatsex.html. Accessed November 6, 1999.

57. Viagra: why aren't more men taking it? *Harvard Health Letter*. October 1999:6.

58. Lue TF. Impotence: a patient's goal-directed approach to treatment. *World J Urol*. 1990;8:67–74.

59. Padma-Nathan H. A new era in the treatment of erectile dysfunction. *Am J Cardiol*. 1999;84:18N–23N.

60. Rosen RC, Cappelleri JC, Smith MD, Lipsky J, Peña BM. Development and evaluation of an abridged, 5-item version of the International Index of Erectile Function (IIEF-5) as a diagnostic tool for erectile dysfunction. *Int J Impot Res*. 1999;11:319–326.

61. Benet AE, Melman A. The epidemiology of erectile dysfunction. *Urol Clin North Am*. 1995;22:699–709.

62. Pritzker MR. The penile stress test: a window to the hearts of man? Abstract presented at: American Heart Association Annual Meeting; November 10, 1999; Atlanta, GA.

63. Impotence may be early warning of heart disease [press release]. Atlanta: Georgia World Congress Center. American Heart Association meeting report; November 10, 1999.

64. Carbone DJ Jr, Harrison LH, McCullough DL. Incidence of previously undiagnosed urologic malignancies in a population presenting solely with the complaint of erectile dysfunction [abstract]. *J Urol*. 1999;161(suppl 4). Abstract 695.

65. Jarow JP, Nana-Sinkam P, Sabbagh M, Eskew A. Outcome analysis of goal directed therapy for impotence. *J Urol*. 1996;155:1609–1612.

66. Jackson G. Erectile dysfunction and cardiovascular disease. *Int J Clin Pract*. 1999;53:363–368.

67. The Process of Care Consensus Panel. The process of care model for evaluation and treatment of erectile dysfunction. *Int J Impot Res*. 1999;11:59–74.

68. Laties AM, Fraunfelder FT. Ocular safety of Viagra, (sildenafil citrate). *Trans Am Ophthalmol Soc*. 1999;97:115–125.

69. Kloner RA, Zusman RM. Cardiovascular effects of sildenafil citrate and recommendations for its use. *Am J Cardiol*. 1999;84:11N–17N.

70. Laudan, L. *Danger Ahead: The Risks You Really Face on Life's Highway*. New York, NY: John Wiley & Sons, Inc; 1997:59,78,116,121,133,152.

71. STATS Statistical Assessment Service. How likely are you to be struck by lightning? Available at: http://www.stats.org/spotlight/2200.html. Accessed December 14, 1999.

72. Muller JE, Mittleman MA, Maclure M, Sherwood JB, Tofler MB, for the Determinants of Myocardial Infarction Onset Study Investigators. Triggering myocardial infarction by sexual activity: low absolute risk and prevention by regular physical exertion. *JAMA*. 1996;275:1405–1409.

73. Walsh, J. *True Odds: How Risk Affects Your Everyday Life*. Los Angeles, CA: Silver Lake Publishing; 1998:9.

74. Singh AD, Paling J. Informed consent: putting risks into perspective. *Survey of Ophthalmology*. 1997;42:83–86.

75. Mittleman MA, Siscovick DS. Physical exertion as a trigger of myocardial infarction and sudden cardiac death. *Cardiol Clin*. 1996;14:263–270.

76. Rosen RC, Leiblum SR. Couples therapy for erectile disorders: observations, obstacles, and outcomes. In: Rosen RC, Leiblum SR, eds. *Erectile Disorders*. New York, NY: The Guilford Press; 1992.

77. Aytac IA, McKinlay JB, Krane RJ. The likely worldwide increase in erectile dysfunction between 1995 and 2025 and some possible policy consequences. *BJU Int*. 1999;84:50–56.

78. Billups K, Friedrich S. Assessment of fasting lipid panels and Doppler ultrasound testing in men presenting with erectile dysfunction and no other medical problems [abstract]. Presented at: American Urological Association Annual Meeting; April 2000; Atlanta, GA. Abstract 655.

79. Men and cardiovascular diseases: biostatistical fact sheets. American Heart Association Web site. Available at: http://www.americanheart.org/statistics/biostats/biome.htm. Accessed on: June 27, 2000.

80. National Library of Medicine Medline search. Available at: http://www.nlm.nih.gov/databases/freemedl.html. Accessed on June 27, 2000.

81. Zippe CD, Jhaveri FM, Klein EA, et al. Role of Viagra after radical prostatectomy. *Urology*. 2000;55:241–245.

82. Weber DC, Bieri S, Kurtz JM, Miralbell R. Prospective pilot study of sildenafil for treatment of postradiotherapy erectile dysfunction in patients with prostate cancer. *J Clin Oncol*. 1999;17:3444–3449.

83. Zelefsky MJ, McKee AB, Lee H, Leibel SA. Efficacy of oral sildenafil in patients with erectile dysfunction after radiotherapy for carcinoma of the prostate. *Urology*. 1999;53:775–778.

84. Merrick GS, Butler WM, Lief JH, Stipetich RL, Abel LJ, Dorsey AT. Efficacy of sildenafil citrate in prostate brachytherapy patients with erectile dysfunction. *Urology*. 1999;53:1112–1116.

85. Kedia S, Zippe CD, Agarwal A, Nelson DR, Lakin MM. Treatment of erectile dysfunction with sildenafil citrate (Viagra) after radiation therapy for prostate cancer. *Urology*. 1999;54:308–312.

86. Jarow JP, Burnett AL, Geringer AM. Clinical efficacy of sildenafil citrate based on etiology and response to prior treatment. *J Urol*. 1999;152:722–725.

87. Virag R, Christiansen E, Guirguis WR, Cox D, Osterloh I. Efficacy of oral sildenafil (Viagra) in a double-blind, placebo-controlled study in men with erectile dysfunction (ED): effect of prior intracavernosal (IC) injection therapy. *J Urol*. 1998;15(suppl).

88. McMahon CG, Samali R, Johnson H. Treatment of intracorporeal injection nonresponse with sildenafil alone or in combination with triple agent intracorporeal injection therapy. *J Urol*. 1999;162:1992–1998.

89. Tur-Kaspa I, Segal S, Moffa F, Massobrio M, Meltzer S. Viagra for temporary erectile dysfunction during treatments with assisted reproductive technologies. *Hum Reprod*. 1999;14:1783–1784.

90. Kaplan B, Ben-Rafael Z, Peled Y, Bar-Hava I, Bar J, Orvieto R. Oral sildenafil may reverse secondary ejaculatory dysfunction during infertility treatment. *Fertil Steril*. 1999;72:1144–1145.

91. Shabsigh R, Klein LT, Seidman S, Kaplan SA, Lehrhoff BJ, Ritter JS. Increased incidence of depressive symptoms in men with erectile dysfunction. *Urology*. 1998;52:848–852.

92. Araujo AB, Durante R, Feldman HA, Goldstein I, McKinlay JB. The relationship between depressive symptoms and male erectile dysfunction: cross-sectional results from the Massachusetts Male Aging Study. *Psychosom Med*. 1998;60:458–465.

93. Thase ME, Reynolds CF III, Jennings JR, et al. Diminished nocturnal penile tumescence in depression: a replication study. *Biol Psychiatry*. 1992;31:1136–1142.

94. Reynolds CF III, Frank E, Thase ME, et al. Assessment of sexual function in depressed, impotent, and healthy men: factor analysis of a brief sexual function questionnaire for men. *Psychiatry Res*. 1988;24:231–250.

95. Menza MA, Roose SP, Seidman SN, et al. Sildenafil citrate for erectile dysfunction and depression [abstract]. Abstracts-On-Disk® of the 1999 APA Annual Meeting; May 19, 1999. Abstract 426.

96. Rosen R, Shabsign R, Menza MA, et al. Sildenafil citrate for erectile dysfunction and depression [abstract]. Abstracts-On-Disk® of the 1999 APA Annual Meeting; May 19, 1999. Abstract 598.

97. Nurnberg HG, Lauriello J, Hensley PL, Parker LM, Keith SJ. Sildenafil for iatrogenic serotonergic antidepressant medication–induced sexual dysfunction in 4 patients. *J Clin Psychiatry*. 1999;60(1):33–35.

98. Fava M, Rankin MA, Alpert JE, Nierenberg AA, Worthington JJ. An open trial of oral sildenafil in antidepressant-induced sexual dysfunction. *Psychother Psychosom*. 1998;67:328–331.

99. Swint S. Viagra may help fight heart failure: two different studies show it has promise [WebMD Medical News Web site]. October 8, 1999. Available at: http://my.webmd.com/content/article/1818.50011. Accessed February 4, 2000.

100. Traverse JH, Du R, Chen YJ, et al. Sildenafil (Viagra) improves coronary blood flow distal to a coronary stenosis during exercise [American Heart Association Abstract Viewer Web site]. November 9, 1999. Available at: http://aha99.agora.com/abstractviewer. Accessed February 15, 2000.

101. Rubin R. First anniversary provides potent cause to celebrate. *USA Today*. March 17, 1999.

SUGGESTED READING ON VIAGRA AND ERECTILE DYSFUNCTION

Cheitlin MD, Hutter AM Jr, Brindis RG, et al. ACC/AHA expert consensus document: use of sildenafil (Viagra) in patients with cardiovascular disease. *J Am Coll Cardiol.* 1999;33:273–282.

Dinsmore WW, Hodges M, Hargreaves C, Osterloh IH, Smith MD, Rosen RC. Sildenafil citrate (Viagra) in erectile dysfunction: near normalization in men with broad spectrum erectile dysfunction compared with age-matched healthy control subjects. *Urology.* 1999; 53:800–805.

Feldman HA, Goldstein I, Hatzichristou DG, Krane RJ, McKinlay JB. Impotence and its medical and psychological correlates: results of the Massachusetts Male Aging Study. *J Urol.* 1994;151:54–61.

Giuliano F, Hultling C, El Masry WS, Smith MD, Osterloh IH, et al. Randomized trial of sildenafil for treatment of erectile dysfunction in spinal injury. Sildenafil Study Group. *Ann Neurol.* 1999;46:15–21.

Goldstein I, Lue TF, Padma-Nathan H, Rosen RC, Steers WD, Wicker PA. Oral sildenafil in the treatment of erectile dysfunction. Sildenafil Study Group. *N Engl J Med.* 1998;338:1397–1404.

Herrmann HC, Chang G, Klugherz BD, Mahoney PD. Hemodynamic effects of sildenafil in men with severe coronary artery disease. *N Engl J Med.* 2000;342: 1622–1626.

Jackson G, Benjamin N, Jackson N, Allen MJ. Effects of sildenafil citrate on human hemodynamics. *Am J Cardiol.* 1999;83:13C–20C.

Jarow JP, Burnett AL, Geringer AM. Clinical efficacy of sildenafil citrate based on etiology and response to prior treatment. *J Urol.* 1999;162:722–725.

Kedia S, Zippe CD, Agarwal A, Nelson DR, Lakin MN. Treatment of erectile dysfunction with sildenafil citrate (Viagra) after radiation therapy for prostate cancer. *Urology.*1999;54:308–312.

Kloner RA, Zusman RM Cardiovascular effects of sildenafil citrate and recommendations for its use. *Am J Cardiol.* 1999;84:11N–17N.

Lue TF. Erectile dysfunction. *N Engl J Med.* 2000; 342:1802–1813.

Maurice WL, Bowman MA. *Sexual Medicine in Primary Care.* St. Louis, MO: Mosby-Year Book; 1998.

Merrick GS, Butler WM, Lief JH, Stipetich RL, Abel LJ, Dorsey AT. Efficacy of sildenafil citrate in prostate brachytherapy patients with erectile dysfunction. *Urology.* 1999;53:1112–1116.

Montorsi F, McDermott TE, Morgan R, et al. Efficacy and safety of fixed-dose oral sildenafil in the treatment of erectile dysfunction of various etiologies. *Urology.* 1999;53:1011–1018.

Morales A, Gingell C, Collins M, Wicker PA, Osterloh IH. Clinical safety of oral sildenafil citrate (VIAGRA) in the treatment of erectile dysfunction. *Int J Impot Res.* 1998;10:69–73.

Padma-Nathan H, Steers WD, Wicker PA. Efficacy and safety of oral sildenafil in the treatment of erectile dysfunction: a double-blind, placebo-controlled study of 329 patients. Sildenafil Study Group. *Int J Clin Pract.* 1998;52:375–379.

Palmer JS, Kaplan WE, Firlit CF. Erectile dysfunction in spina bifida is treatable. *Lancet.* 1999;354:125–126.

Rendell MS, Rajfer J, Wicker PA, Smith MD. Sildenafil for treatment of erectile dysfunction in men with diabetes: a randomized controlled trial. Sildenafil Diabetes Study Group. *JAMA.* 1999;281:421–426.

Steers WD. Viagra—after one year. *Urology.* 1999;54: 12–17.

Weber DC, Bieri S, Kurtz JM, Miralbell R. Prospective pilot study of sildenafil for treatment of postradiotherapy erectile dysfunction in patients with prostate cancer. *J Clin Oncol.* 1999;17:3444–3449.

Zippe CD, Jhaveri FM, Klein EA, et al. Role of Viagra after radical prostatectomy. *Urology.* 2000;55:241–245.

Zusman RM, Morales A, Glasser DB, Osterloh IH. Overall cardiovascular profile of sildenafil citrate. *Am J Cardiol.* 1999;83:35C–44C.

INDEX

FIGURE ACKNOWLEDGMENTS

The Publisher acknowledges the following individuals and companies for illustrations, graphs, and tables appearing on the pages noted below:

Chapter 1:

Opening spread: Private Collection
Page 2 (painting): © Bettman/CORBIS
Page 2 (book): © Phil Schermeister, AllStock/ PictureQuest
Page 6 (Dr. Brindley): David Montgomery at M+M Management
Page 6 (syringe): Digital imagery® copyright 1999 PhotoDisc, Inc.
Pages 6–7 (cassette): © PhotoDisc, Inc.
Page 7, top and bottom 3 drawings: © 1999 Photographs provided courtesy of the National Foundation for Sexual Health Medicine, Inc., formerly known as the National Erectile Dysfunction Foundation, Inc. All rights reserved.
Page 7 (surgeon photo): © PhotoDisc, Inc.

Chapter 2:

Page 13 (graph): Reprinted from *American Journal of Cardiology*, Vol. 83, David J. Webb, Stephen Freestone, Michael J. Allen, Gary J. Muirhead, Sildenafil citrate and blood-pressure-lowering drugs: results of drug interaction studies with an organic nitrate and a calcium antagonist, p. 21C–28C, © 1999, with permission from Excerpta Medica Inc.
Page 14 (Dr. Rajfer): Courtesy of Jacob Rajfer, MD, Los Angeles, California
Page 14 (elevator door): © Nathan Benn/Stock, Boston
Page 15 (RigiScan): Courtesy of Laurence Levine, MD, Chicago, Illinois
Page 16 (graph): Reprinted from *British Journal of Urology*, Vol. 78, M. Boolell, S. Gepi-Attee, J.C. Gingell, M.J. Allen, Sildenafil, a novel effective oral therapy for male erectile dysfunction, p. 257-261, © 1996, with permission.
Page 16 (stopwatch): © Paramount/Viacom/ PictureQuest

Chapter 3:

Opening spread (Dr. Ignarro receiving Nobel prize) and page 20 (top): Kean/Archive Photos
Opening spread and page 21(cover of Science): Reprinted with permission from *Science*, Vol. 258, December 18, 1992. Copyright 1992 American Association for the Advancement of Science.
Opening spread and page 21(cover of Science, nitric oxide image): Visuals Unlimited, Inc.
Page 21 (Dr. Ignarro): Courtesy of Louis J. Ignarro, PhD., Los Angeles, California
Page 25, bottom (table): Adapted from *American Journal of Cardiology*, Vol. 83, Robert M. Wallis, Jackie D. Corbin, Sharron H. Francis, Peter Ellis, Tissue distribution of phosphodiesterase families and the effects of sildenafil on tissue cyclic nucleotides, platelet function, and the contractile responses of trabeculae carneae and aortic rings in vitro, p. 3C–12C, ©1999, with permission from Excerpta Medica Inc.

Chapter 4:

Page 28 (Dr. Rosen): New Jersey Newsphotos, Newark, New Jersey
Page 29, entire page (IIEF, also on page 27): Reprinted from *Urology*, Vol. 49, No. 6, Raymond C. Rosen, Alan Riley, Gorm Wagner, Ian H. Osterloh, John Kirkpatrick, Avanish Mishra, The international index of erectile function (IIEF): a multidimensional scale for assessment of erectile dysfunction, p. 822–830, 1997, with permission from Elsevier Science.
Page 30 (blackboard, composition book): © PhotoDisc, Inc.
Page 32 (Dr. Cox): Courtesy of Dr. David Cox, Kent, England
Page 32 (phone receiver): © PhotoDisc, Inc.
Page 33 (man and woman): © Anthony Nagleman/ FPG International LLC
Page 36, top (graph): Reprinted from *American Journal of Cardiology*, Vol. 83, No. 5A, Randall M. Zusman, Alvaro Morales, Dale B. Glasser, Ian H. Osterloh, Overall cardiovascular profile of sildenafil citrate, p. 35C–44C, © 1999, with permission from Excerpta Medica Inc.
Page 36, bottom (graph): From *International Journal of Clinical Practice*, Vol. 52, No. 6, H. Padma-Nathan, W.D. Steers, P.A. Wicker, Efficacy and safety of oral sildenafil in the treatment of erectile dysfunction: a double-blind, placebo-controlled study of 329 patients, p. 375–380, 1998.
Page 37 (journal cover): Copyright © 1998 Massachusetts Medical Society. Reproduced by permission. All rights reserved. This cover and page of the *Journal* may not be further reproduced without the express written permission of the copyright owner. Contact: Rights & Permissions Dept., Publishing Div. of the MMS, 860 Winter Street, Waltham, MA 02451-1413 USA.

Chapter 5:

Page 45 (telegraph office): © Archive Photos/ Herbert Photography
Page 46 (peace sign): © PhotoDisc, Inc.
Page 47 (magazine cover): © 1997 Newsweek, Inc. All rights reserved. Reprinted by permission.
Page 47 (magazine cover, pill image): Oskar Martinez
Page 48 (hand with magnifying glass): ©PhotoDisc, Inc.
Page 52 (Dr. Sadovsky): © 1999 Photograph provided courtesy of the National Foundation for Sexual Health Medicine, Inc., formerly known as the National Erectile Dysfunction Foundation, Inc. All rights reserved.

(continues)

VIAGRA®
(sildenafil citrate)
Tablets

DESCRIPTION

VIAGRA®, an oral therapy for erectile dysfunction, is the citrate salt of sildenafil, a selective inhibitor of cyclic guanosine monophosphate (cGMP)-specific phosphodiesterase type 5 (PDE5).

Sildenafil citrate is designated chemically as 1-[[3-(6,7-dihydro-1-methyl-7-oxo-3-propyl-1*H*-pyrazolo[4,3-*d*]pyrimidin-5-yl)-4-ethoxyphenyl]sulfonyl]-4-methyl-piperazine citrate and has the following structural formula:

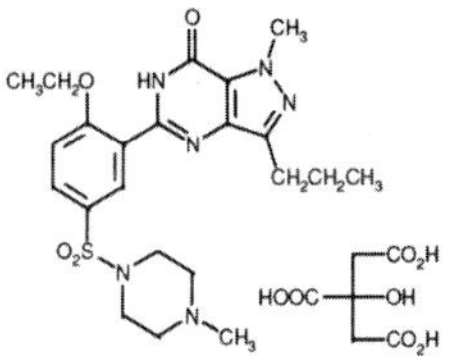

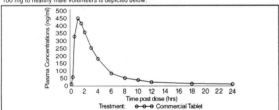

Sildenafil citrate is a white to off-white crystalline powder with a solubility of 3.5 mg/mL in water and a molecular weight of 666.7. VIAGRA (sildenafil citrate) is formulated as blue, film-coated rounded-diamond-shaped tablets equivalent to 25 mg, 50 mg and 100 mg of sildenafil for oral administration. In addition to the active ingredient, sildenafil citrate, each tablet contains the following inactive ingredients: microcrystalline cellulose, anhydrous dibasic calcium phosphate, croscarmellose sodium, magnesium stearate, hydroxypropyl methylcellulose, titanium dioxide, lactose, triacetin, and FD & C Blue #2 aluminum lake.

CLINICAL PHARMACOLOGY

Mechanism of Action

The physiologic mechanism of erection of the penis involves release of nitric oxide (NO) in the corpus cavernosum during sexual stimulation. NO then activates the enzyme guanylate cyclase, which results in increased levels of cyclic guanosine monophosphate (cGMP), producing smooth muscle relaxation in the corpus cavernosum and allowing inflow of blood. Sildenafil has no direct relaxant effect on isolated human corpus cavernosum, but enhances the effect of nitric oxide (NO) by inhibiting phosphodiesterase type 5 (PDE5), which is responsible for degradation of cGMP in the corpus cavernosum. When sexual stimulation causes local release of NO, inhibition of PDE5 by sildenafil causes increased levels of cGMP in the corpus cavernosum, resulting in smooth muscle relaxation and inflow of blood to the corpus cavernosum. Sildenafil at recommended doses has no effect in the absence of sexual stimulation.

Studies *in vitro* have shown that sildenafil is selective for PDE5. Its effect is more potent on PDE5 than on other known phosphodiesterases (>80-fold for PDE1, >1,000-fold for PDE2, PDE3, and PDE4). The approximately 4,000-fold selectivity for PDE5 versus PDE3 is important because that PDE is involved in control of cardiac contractility. Sildenafil is only about 10-fold as potent for PDE5 compared to PDE6, an enzyme found in the retina; this lower selectivity is thought to be the basis for abnormalities related to color vision observed with higher doses or plasma levels (see **Pharmacodynamics**).

In addition to human corpus cavernosum smooth muscle, PDE5 is also found in lower concentrations in other tissues including platelets, vascular and visceral smooth muscle, and skeletal muscle. The inhibition of PDE5 in these tissues by sildenafil may be the basis for the enhanced platelet antiaggregatory activity of nitric oxide observed *in vitro*, an inhibition of platelet thrombus formation *in vivo* and peripheral arterial-venous dilatation *in vivo*.

Pharmacokinetics and Metabolism

VIAGRA is rapidly absorbed after oral administration, with absolute bioavailability of about 40%. Its pharmacokinetics are dose-proportional over the recommended dose range. It is eliminated predominantly by hepatic metabolism (mainly cytochrome P450 3A4) and is converted to an active metabolite with properties similar to the parent, sildenafil. The concomitant use of potent cytochrome P450 3A4 inhibitors (e.g., erythromycin, ketoconazole, itraconazole) as well as the nonspecific CYP inhibitor, cimetidine, is associated with increased plasma levels of sildenafil (see **DOSAGE AND ADMINISTRATION**). Both sildenafil and the metabolite have terminal half lives of about 4 hours.

Mean sildenafil plasma concentrations measured after the administration of a single oral dose of 100 mg to healthy male volunteers is depicted below:

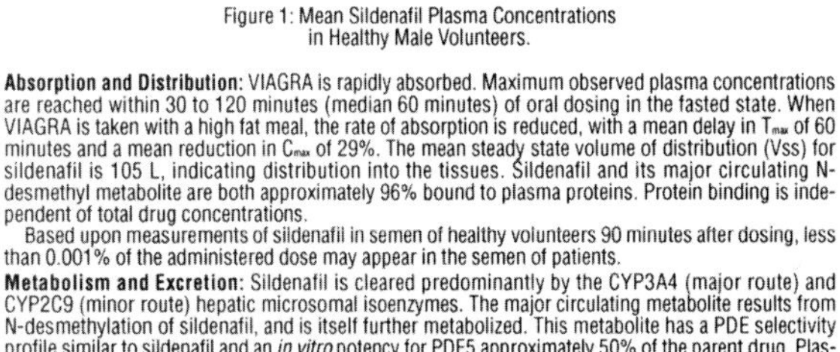

Figure 1: Mean Sildenafil Plasma Concentrations in Healthy Male Volunteers.

Absorption and Distribution: VIAGRA is rapidly absorbed. Maximum observed plasma concentrations are reached within 30 to 120 minutes (median 60 minutes) of oral dosing in the fasted state. When VIAGRA is taken with a high fat meal, the rate of absorption is reduced, with a mean delay in T_{max} of 60 minutes and a mean reduction in C_{max} of 29%. The mean steady state volume of distribution (Vss) for sildenafil is 105 L, indicating distribution into the tissues. Sildenafil and its major circulating N-desmethyl metabolite are both approximately 96% bound to plasma proteins. Protein binding is independent of total drug concentrations.

Based upon measurements of sildenafil in semen of healthy volunteers 90 minutes after dosing, less than 0.001% of the administered dose may appear in the semen of patients.

Metabolism and Excretion: Sildenafil is cleared predominantly by the CYP3A4 (major route) and CYP2C9 (minor route) hepatic microsomal isoenzymes. The major circulating metabolite results from N-desmethylation of sildenafil, and is itself further metabolized. This metabolite has a PDE selectivity profile similar to sildenafil and an *in vitro* potency for PDE5 approximately 50% of the parent drug. Plasma concentrations of this metabolite are approximately 40% of those seen for sildenafil, so that the metabolite accounts for about 20% of sildenafil's pharmacologic effects.

After either oral or intravenous administration, sildenafil is excreted as metabolites predominantly in the feces (approximately 80% of administered oral dose) and to a lesser extent in the urine (approximately 13% of the administered oral dose). Similar values for pharmacokinetic parameters were seen in normal volunteers and in the patient population, using a population pharmacokinetic approach.

Pharmacokinetics in Special Populations

Geriatrics: Healthy elderly volunteers (65 years or over) had a reduced clearance of sildenafil, with free plasma concentrations approximately 40% greater than those seen in healthy younger volunteers (18-45 years).

Renal Insufficiency: In volunteers with mild (CLcr = 50-80 mL/min) and moderate (CLcr = 30-49 mL/min) renal impairment, the pharmacokinetics of a single oral dose of VIAGRA (50 mg) were not altered. In volunteers with severe (CLcr = <30 mL/min) renal impairment, sildenafil clearance was reduced, resulting in approximately doubling of AUC and C_{max} compared to age-matched volunteers with no renal impairment.

Hepatic Insufficiency: In volunteers with hepatic cirrhosis (Child-Pugh A and B), sildenafil clearance was reduced, resulting in increases in AUC (84%) and C_{max} (47%) compared to age-matched volunteers with no hepatic impairment.

Therefore, age>65, hepatic impairment and severe renal impairment are associated with increased plasma levels of sildenafil. A starting oral dose of 25 mg should be considered in those patients (see **DOSAGE AND ADMINISTRATION**).

Pharmacodynamics

Effects of VIAGRA on Erectile Response: In eight double-blind, placebo-controlled crossover studies of patients with either organic or psychogenic erectile dysfunction, sexual stimulation resulted in improved erections, as assessed by an objective measurement of hardness and duration of erections (RigiScan®), after VIAGRA administration compared with placebo. Most studies assessed the efficacy of VIAGRA approximately 60 minutes post dose. The erectile response, as assessed by RigiScan®, generally increased with increasing sildenafil dose and plasma concentration. The time course of effect was examined in one study, showing an effect for up to 4 hours but the response was diminished compared to 2 hours.

Effects of VIAGRA on Blood Pressure: Single oral doses of sildenafil (100 mg) administered to healthy volunteers produced decreases in supine blood pressure (mean maximum decrease of 8.4/5.5 mmHg). The decrease in blood pressure was most notable approximately 1-2 hours after dosing, and was not different than placebo at 8 hours. Similar effects on blood pressure were noted with 25 mg, 50 mg and 100 mg of VIAGRA, therefore the effects are not related to dose or plasma levels. Larger effects were recorded among patients receiving concomitant nitrates (see **CONTRAINDICATIONS**).

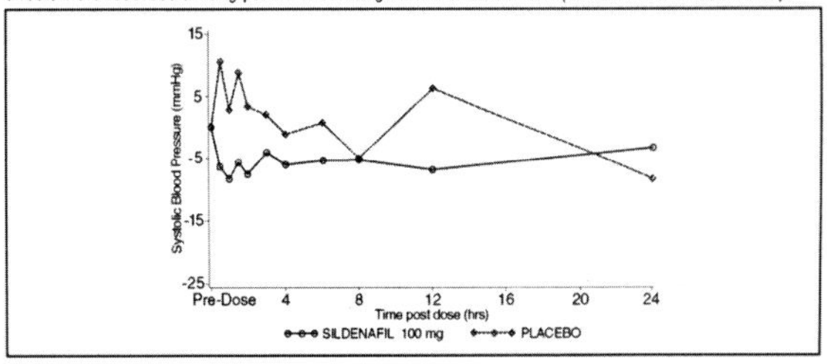

Figure 2: Mean Change from Baseline in Sitting Systolic Blood Pressure, Healthy Volunteers.

Effects of VIAGRA on Cardiac Parameters: Single oral doses of sildenafil up to 100 mg produced no clinically relevant changes in the ECGs of normal male volunteers.

Studies have produced relevant data on the effects of VIAGRA on cardiac output. In one small, open-label, uncontrolled, pilot study, eight patients with stable ischemic heart disease underwent Swan-Ganz catheterization. A total dose of 40 mg sildenafil was administered by four intravenous infusions.

The results from this pilot study are shown in Table 1; the mean resting systolic and diastolic blood pressures decreased by 7% and 10% compared to baseline in these patients. Mean resting values for right atrial pressure, pulmonary artery pressure, pulmonary artery occluded pressure and cardiac output decreased by 28%, 28%, 20% and 7% respectively. Even though this total dosage produced plasma sildenafil concentrations which were approximately 2 to 5 times higher than the mean maximum plasma concentrations following a single oral dose of 100 mg in healthy male volunteers, the hemodynamic response to exercise was preserved in these patients.

TABLE 1. HEMODYNAMIC DATA IN PATIENTS WITH STABLE ISCHEMIC HEART DISEASE AFTER IV ADMINISTRATION OF 40 MG SILDENAFIL

Means ± SD	At rest			
	n	Baseline (B2)	n	Sildenafil (D1)
PAOP (mmHg)	8	8.1 ± 5.1	8	6.5 ± 4.3
Mean PAP (mmHg)	8	16.7 ± 4	8	12.1 ± 3.9
Mean RAP (mmHg)	7	5.7 ± 3.7	8	4.1 ± 3.7
Systolic SAP (mmHg)	8	150.4 ± 12.4	8	140.6 ± 16.5
Diastolic SAP (mmHg)	8	73.6 ± 7.8	8	65.9 ± 10
Cardiac output (L/min)	8	5.6 ± 0.9	8	5.2 ± 1.1
Heart rate (bpm)	8	67 ± 11.1	8	66.9 ± 12
Means ± SD	**After 4 minutes of exercise**			
	n	Baseline	n	Sildenafil
PAOP (mmHg)	8	36.0 ± 13.7	8	27.8 ± 15.3
Mean PAP (mmHg)	8	39.4 ± 12.9	8	31.7 ± 13.2
Mean RAP (mmHg)	-	-	-	-
Systolic SAP (mmHg)	8	199.5 ± 37.4	8	187.8 ± 30.0
Diastolic SAP (mmHg)	8	84.6 ± 9.7	8	79.5 ± 9.4
Cardiac output (L/min)	8	11.5 ± 2.4	8	10.2 ± 3.5
Heart rate (bpm)	8	101.9 ± 11.6	8	99.0 ± 20.4

Effects of VIAGRA on Vision: At single oral doses of 100 mg and 200 mg, transient dose-related impairment of color discrimination (blue/green) was detected using the Farnsworth-Munsell 100-hue test, with peak effects near the time of peak plasma levels. This finding is consistent with the inhibition of PDE6, which is involved in phototransduction in the retina. An evaluation of visual function at doses up to twice the maximum recommended dose revealed no effects of VIAGRAon visual acuity, intraocular pressure, or pupillometry.

Clinical Studies

In clinical studies, VIAGRA was assessed for its effect on the ability of men with erectile dysfunction (ED) to engage in sexual activity and in many cases specifically on the ability to achieve and maintain an erection sufficient for satisfactory sexual activity. VIAGRA was evaluated primarily at doses of 25 mg, 50 mg and 100 mg in 21 randomized, double-blind, placebo-controlled trials of up to 6 months in duration, using a variety of study designs (fixed dose, titration, parallel, crossover). VIAGRA was administered to more than 3,000 patients aged 19 to 87 years, with ED of various etiologies (organic, psychogenic, mixed) with a mean duration of 5 years. VIAGRA demonstrated statistically significant improvement compared to placebo in all 21 studies. The studies that established benefit demonstrated improvements in success rates for sexual intercourse compared with placebo.

The effectiveness of VIAGRA was evaluated in most studies using several assessment instruments. The primary measure in the principal studies was a sexual function questionnaire (the International Index of Erectile Function - IIEF) administered during a 4-week treatment-free run-in period, at baseline, at follow-up visits, and at the end of double-blind, placebo-controlled, at-home treatment. Two of the questions from the IIEF served as primary study endpoints; categorical responses were elicited to questions about (1) the ability to achieve erections sufficient for sexual intercourse and (2) the maintenance of erections after penetration. The patient addressed both questions at the final visit for the last 4 weeks of the study. The possible categorical responses to these questions were (0) no attempted intercourse, (1) never or almost never, (2) a few times, (3) sometimes, (4) most times, and (5) almost always or always. Also collected as part of the IIEF was information about other aspects of sexual function, including information on erectile function, orgasm, desire, satisfaction with intercourse, and overall sexual satisfaction. Sexual function data were also recorded by patients in a daily diary. In addition, patients were asked a global efficacy question and an optional partner questionnaire was administered.

The effect on one of the major end points, maintenance of erections after penetration, is shown in Figure 3, for the pooled results of 5 fixed-dose, dose-response studies of greater than one month duration, showing response according to baseline function. Results with all doses have been pooled, but scores showed greater improvement at the 50 and 100 mg doses than at 25 mg. The pattern of responses was similar for the other principal question, the ability to achieve an erection sufficient for intercourse. The titration studies, in which most patients received 100 mg, showed similar results. Figure 3 shows that regardless of the baseline levels of function, subsequent function in patients treated with VIAGRA was better than that seen in patients treated with placebo. At the same time, on-treatment function was better in treated patients who were less impaired at baseline.

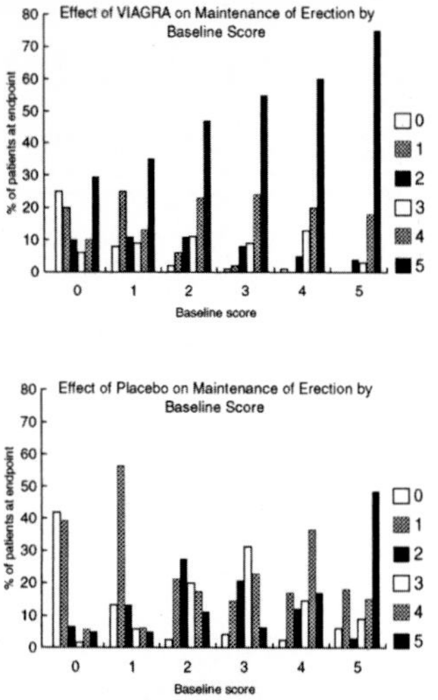

Figure 3. Effect of VIAGRA and Placebo on Maintenance of Erection by Baseline Score.

The frequency of patients reporting improvement of erections in response to a global question in four of the randomized, double-blind, parallel, placebo-controlled fixed dose studies (1797 patients) of 12 to 24 weeks duration is shown in Figure 4. These patients had erectile dysfunction at baseline that was characterized by median categorical scores of 2 (a few times) on principal IIEF questions. Erectile dysfunction was attributed to organic (58%; generally not characterized, but including diabetes and excluding spinal cord injury), psychogenic (17%), or mixed (24%) etiologies. Sixty-three percent, 74%, and 82% of the patients on 25 mg, 50 mg and 100 mg of VIAGRA, respectively, reported an improvement in their erections, compared to 24% on placebo. In the titration studies (n=644) (with most patients eventually receiving 100 mg), results were similar.

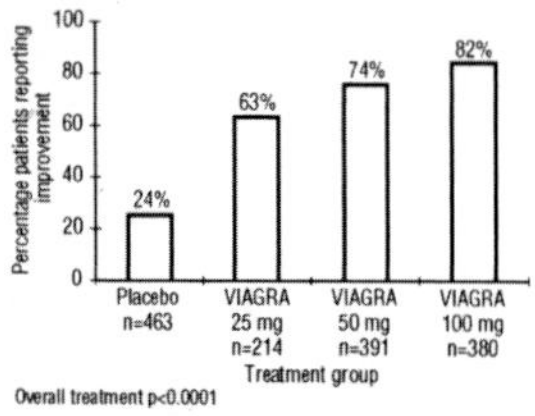

Figure 4. Percentage of Patients Reporting an Improvement in Erections.

The patients in studies had varying degrees of ED. One-third to one-half of the subjects in these studies reported successful intercourse at least once during a 4-week, treatment-free run-in period.

In many of the studies, of both fixed dose and titration designs, daily diaries were kept by patients. In these studies, involving about 1600 patients, analyses of patient diaries showed no effect of VIAGRA on rates of attempted intercourse (about 2 per week), but there was clear treatment-related improvement in sexual function: per patient weekly success rates averaged 1.3 on 50-100 mg of VIAGRA vs 0.4 on placebo; similarly, group mean success rates (total successes divided by total attempts) were about 66% on VIAGRA vs about 20% on placebo.

During 3 to 6 months of double-blind treatment or longer-term (1 year), open-label studies, few patients withdrew from active treatment for any reason, including lack of effectiveness. At the end of the long-term study, 88% of patients reported that VIAGRA improved their erections.

Men with untreated ED had relatively low baseline scores for all aspects of sexual function measured (again using a 5-point scale) in the IIEF. VIAGRA improved these aspects of sexual function: frequency, firmness and maintenance of erections; frequency of orgasm; frequency and level of desire; frequency, satisfaction and enjoyment of intercourse; and overall relationship satisfaction.

One randomized, double-blind, flexible-dose, placebo-controlled study included only patients with erectile dysfunction attributed to complications of diabetes mellitus (n=268). As in the other titration studies, patients were started on 50 mg and allowed to adjust the dose up to 100 mg or down to 25 mg of VIAGRA; all patients, however, were receiving 50 mg or 100 mg at the end of the study. There were highly statistically significant improvements on the two principal IIEF questions (frequency of successful penetration during sexual activity and maintenance of erections after penetration) on VIAGRA compared to placebo. On a global improvement question, 57% of VIAGRA patients reported improved erections versus 10% on placebo. Diary data indicated that on VIAGRA, 48% of intercourse attempts were successful versus 12% on placebo.

One randomized, double-blind, placebo-controlled, crossover, flexible-dose (up to 100 mg) study of patients with erectile dysfunction resulting from spinal cord injury (n=178) was conducted. The changes from baseline in scoring on the two end point questions (frequency of successful penetration during sexual activity and maintenance of erections after penetration) were highly statistically significantly in favor of VIAGRA. On a global improvement question, 83% of patients reported improved erections on VIAGRA versus 12% on placebo. Diary data indicated that on VIAGRA, 59% of attempts at sexual intercourse were successful compared to 13% on placebo.

Across all trials, VIAGRA improved the erections of 43% of radical prostatectomy patients compared to 15% on placebo.

Subgroup analyses of responses to a global improvement question in patients with psychogenic etiology in two fixed-dose studies (total n=179) and two titration studies (total n=149) showed 84% of VIAGRA patients reported improvement in erections compared with 26% of placebo. The changes from baseline in scoring on the two end point questions (frequency of successful penetration during sexual activity and maintenance of erections after penetration) were highly statistically significantly in favor of VIAGRA. Diary data in two of the studies (n=178) showed rates of successful intercourse per attempt of 70% for VIAGRA and 29% for placebo.

A review of population subgroups demonstrated efficacy regardless of baseline severity, etiology, race and age. VIAGRA was effective in a broad range of ED patients, including those with a history of coronary artery disease, hypertension, other cardiac disease, peripheral vascular disease, diabetes mellitus, depression, coronary artery bypass graft (CABG), radical prostatectomy, transurethral resection of the prostate (TURP) and spinal cord injury, and in patients taking antidepressants/antipsychotics and antihypertensives/diuretics.

Analysis of the safety database showed no apparent difference in the side effect profile in patients taking VIAGRA with and without antihypertensive medication. This analysis was performed retrospectively, and was not powered to detect any pre-specified difference in adverse reactions.

INDICATION AND USAGE

VIAGRA is indicated for the treatment of erectile dysfunction.

CONTRAINDICATIONS

Consistent with its known effects on the nitric oxide/cGMP pathway (see **CLINICAL PHARMACOLOGY**), VIAGRA was shown to potentiate the hypotensive effects of nitrates, and its administration to patients who are using organic nitrates, either regularly and/or intermittently, in any form is therefore contraindicated.

After patients have taken VIAGRA, it is unknown when nitrates, if necessary, can be safely administered. Based on the pharmacokinetic profile of a single 100 mg oral dose given to healthy normal volunteers, the plasma levels of sildenafil at 24 hours post dose are approximately 2 ng/mL (compared to peak plasma levels of approximately 440 ng/mL) (see **CLINICAL PHARMACOLOGY: Pharmacokinetics and Metabolism**). In the following patients: age>65, hepatic impairment (e.g., cirrhosis), severe renal impairment (e.g., creatinine clearance <30 mL/min), and concomitant use of potent cytochrome P450 3A4 inhibitors (erythromycin), plasma levels of sildenafil at 24 hours post dose have been found to be 3 to 8 times higher than those seen in healthy volunteers. Although plasma levels of sildenafil at 24 hours post dose are much lower than at peak concentration, it is unknown whether nitrates can be safely coadministered at this time point.

VIAGRA is contraindicated in patients with a known hypersensitivity to any component of the tablet.

WARNINGS

There is a potential for cardiac risk of sexual activity in patients with preexisting cardiovascular disease. Therefore, treatments for erectile dysfunction, including VIAGRA, should not be generally used in men for whom sexual activity is inadvisable because of their underlying cardiovascular status.

VIAGRA has systemic vasodilatory properties that resulted in transient decreases in supine blood pressure in healthy volunteers (mean maximum decrease of 8.4/5.5 mmHg), (see **CLINICAL PHARMACOLOGY: Pharmacodynamics**). While this normally would be expected to be of little consequence in most patients, prior to prescribing VIAGRA, physicians should carefully consider whether their patients with underlying cardiovascular disease could be affected adversely by such vasodilatory effects, especially in combination with sexual activity.

There is no controlled clinical data on the safety or efficacy of VIAGRA in the following groups; if prescribed, this should be done with caution.

- Patients who have suffered a myocardial infarction, stroke, or life-threatening arrhythmia within the last 6 months;
- Patients with resting hypotension (BP <90/50) or hypertension (BP >170/110);
- Patients with cardiac failure or coronary artery disease causing unstable angina;
- Patients with retinitis pigmentosa (a minority of these patients have genetic disorders of retinal phosphodiesterases).

Prolonged erection greater than 4 hours and priapism (painful erections greater than 6 hours in duration) have been reported infrequently since market approval of VIAGRA. In the event of an erection that persists longer than 4 hours, the patient should seek immediate medical assistance. If priapism is not treated immediately, penile tissue damage and permanent loss of potency could result.

The concomitant administration of the protease inhibitor ritonavir substantially increases serum concentrations of sildenafil (**11-fold increase in AUC**). If VIAGRA is prescribed to patients taking ritonavir, caution should be used. Data from subjects exposed to high systemic levels of sildenafil are limited. Visual disturbances occurred more commonly at higher levels of sildenafil exposure. Decreased blood pressure, syncope, and prolonged erection were reported in some healthy volunteers exposed to high doses of sildenafil (200-800 mg). To decrease the chance of adverse events in patients taking ritonavir, a decrease in sildenafil dosage is recommended (see **Drug Interactions, ADVERSE REACTIONS** and **DOSAGE AND ADMINISTRATION**).

PRECAUTIONS

General

The evaluation of erectile dysfunction should include a determination of potential underlying causes and the identification of appropriate treatment following a complete medical assessment.

Before prescribing VIAGRA, it is important to note the following:

Patients on multiple antihypertensive medications were included in the pivotal clinical trials for VIAGRA. In a separate drug interaction study, when amlodipine, 5 mg or 10 mg, and VIAGRA, 100 mg were orally administered concomitantly to hypertensive patients mean additional blood pressure reduction of 8 mmHg systolic and 7 mmHg dia-stolic were noted (see **Drug Interactions**). Controlled studies of drug interactions between VIAGRA and other antihypertensive medications have not been performed.

The safety of VIAGRA is unknown in patients with bleeding disorders and patients with active peptic ulceration.

VIAGRA should be used with caution in patients with anatomical deformation of the penis (such as angulation, cavernosal fibrosis or Peyronie's disease), or in patients who have conditions which may predispose them to priapism (such as sickle cell anemia, multiple myeloma, or leukemia).

The safety and efficacy of combinations of VIAGRA with other treatments for erectile dysfunction have not been studied. Therefore, the use of such combinations is not recommended.

In humans, VIAGRA has no effect on bleeding time when taken alone or with aspirin. *In vitro* studies with human platelets indicate that sildenafil potentiates the antiaggregatory effect of sodium nitroprusside (a nitric oxide donor). The combination of heparin and VIAGRA had an additive effect on bleeding time in the anesthetized rabbit, but this interaction has not been studied in humans.

Information for Patients

Physicians should discuss with patients the contraindication of VIAGRA with regular and/or intermittent use of organic nitrates.

Physicians should discuss with patients the potential cardiac risk of sexual activity in patients with preexisting cardiovascular risk factors. Patients who experience symptoms (e.g., angina pectoris, dizziness, nausea) upon initiation of sexual activity should be advised to refrain from further activity and should discuss the episode with their physician.

Physicians should warn patients that prolonged erections greater than 4 hours and priapism (painful erections greater than 6 hours in duration) have been reported infrequently since market approval of VIAGRA. In the event of an erection that persists longer than 4 hours, the patient should seek immediate medical assistance. If priapism is not treated immediately, penile tissue damage and permanent loss of potency may result.

The use of VIAGRA offers no protection against sexually transmitted diseases. Counseling of patients about the protective measures necessary to guard against sexually transmitted diseases, including the Human Immunodeficiency Virus (HIV), may be considered.

Drug Interactions

Effects of Other Drugs on VIAGRA

***In vitro* studies:** Sildenafil metabolism is principally mediated by the cytochrome P450 (CYP) isoforms 3A4 (major route) and 2C9 (minor route). Therefore, inhibitors of these isoenzymes may reduce sildenafil clearance.

***In vivo* studies:** Cimetidine (800 mg), a nonspecific CYP inhibitor, caused a 56% increase in plasma sildenafil concentrations when coadministered with VIAGRA (50 mg) to healthy volunteers.

When a single 100 mg dose of VIAGRA was administered with erythromycin, a specific CYP3A4 inhibitor, at steady state (500 mg bid for 5 days), there was a 182% increase in sildenafil systemic exposure (AUC). In addition, in a study performed in healthy male volunteers, coadministration of the HIV protease inhibitor saquinavir, also a CYP3A4 inhibitor, at steady state (1200 mg tid) with VIAGRA (100 mg single dose) resulted in a 140% increase in sildenafil C_{max} and a 210% increase in sildenafil AUC. VIAGRA had no effect on saquinavir pharmacokinetics. Stronger CYP3A4 inhibitors such as ketoconazole or itraconazole would be expected to have still greater effects, and population data from patients in clinical trials did indicate a reduction in sildenafil clearance when it was coadministered with CYP3A4 inhibitors (such as ketoconazole, erythromycin, or cimetidine) (see **DOSAGE AND ADMINISTRATION**).

In another study in healthy male volunteers, coadministration with the HIV protease inhibitor ritonavir, which is a highly potent P450 inhibitor, at steady state (500 mg bid) with VIAGRA (100 mg single dose) resulted in a 300% (4-fold) increase in sildenafil C_{max} and a 1000% (11-fold) increase in sildenafil plasma AUC. At 24 hours the plasma levels of sildenafil were still approximately 200 ng/mL, compared to approximately 5 ng/mL when sildenafil was dosed alone. This is consistent with ritonavir's marked effects on a broad range of P450 substrates. VIAGRA had no effect on ritonavir pharmacokinetics (see **DOSAGE AND ADMINISTRATION**).

Although the interaction between other protease inhibitors and sildenafil has not been studied, their concomitant use is expected to increase sildenafil levels.

It can be expected that concomitant administration of CYP3A4 inducers, such as rifampin, will decrease plasma levels of sildenafil.

Single doses of antacid (magnesium hydroxide/aluminum hydroxide) did not affect the bioavailability of VIAGRA.

Pharmacokinetic data from patients in clinical trials showed no effect on sildenafil pharmacokinetics of CYP2C9 inhibitors (such as tolbutamide, warfarin), CYP2D6 inhibitors (such as selective serotonin reuptake inhibitors, tricyclic antidepressants, thiazide and related diuretics, ACE inhibitors, and calcium channel blockers. The AUC of the active metabolite, N-desmethyl sildenafil, was increased 62% by loop and potassium-sparing diuretics and 102% by nonspecific beta-blockers. These effects on the metabolite are not expected to be of clinical consequence.

Effects of VIAGRA on Other Drugs
In vitro studies: Sildenafil is a weak inhibitor of the cytochrome P450 isoforms 1A2, 2C9, 2C19, 2D6, 2E1 and 3A4 (IC50 >150 µM). Given sildenafil peak plasma concentrations of approximately 1 µM after recommended doses, it is unlikely that VIAGRA will alter the clearance of substrates of these isoenzymes.

In vivo studies: When VIAGRA 100 mg oral was coadministered with amlodipine, 5 mg or 10 mg oral, to hypertensive patients, the mean additional reduction on supine blood pressure was 8 mmHg systolic and 7 mmHg diastolic.

No significant interactions were shown with tolbutamide (250 mg) or warfarin (40 mg), both of which are metabolized by CYP2C9.

VIAGRA (50 mg) did not potentiate the increase in bleeding time caused by aspirin (150 mg).

VIAGRA (50 mg) did not potentiate the hypotensive effect of alcohol in healthy volunteers with mean maximum blood alcohol levels of 0.08%.

In a study of healthy male volunteers, sildenafil (100 mg) did not affect the steady state pharmacokinetics of the HIV protease inhibitors, saquinavir and ritonavir, both of which are CYP3A4 substrates.

Carcinogenesis, Mutagenesis, Impairment of Fertility
Sildenafil was not carcinogenic when administered to rats for 24 months at a dose resulting in total systemic drug exposure (AUCs) for unbound sildenafil and its major metabolite of 29- and 42-times, for male and female rats, respectively, the exposures observed in human males given the Maximum Recommended Human Dose (MRHD) of 100 mg. Sildenafil was not carcinogenic when administered to mice for 18-21 months at dosages up to the Maximum Tolerated Dose (MTD) of 10 mg/kg/day, approximately 0.6 times the MRHD on a mg/m² basis.

Sildenafil was negative in *in vitro* bacterial and Chinese hamster ovary cell assays to detect mutagenicity, and *in vitro* human lymphocytes and *in vivo* mouse micronucleus assays to detect clastogenicity.

There was no impairment of fertility in rats given sildenafil up to 60 mg/kg/day for 36 days to females and 102 days to males, a dose producing an AUC value of more than 25 times the human male AUC.

There was no effect on sperm motility or morphology after single 100 mg oral doses of VIAGRA in healthy volunteers.

Pregnancy, Nursing Mothers and Pediatric Use
VIAGRA is not indicated for use in newborns, children, or women.

Pregnancy Category B. No evidence of teratogenicity, embryotoxicity or fetotoxicity was observed in rats and rabbits which received up to 200 mg/kg/day during organogenesis. These doses represent, respectively, about 20 and 40 times the MRHD on a mg/m² basis in a 50 kg subject. In the rat pre- and postnatal development study, the no observed adverse effect dose was 30 mg/kg/day given for 36 days. In the nonpregnant rat the AUC at this dose was about 20 times human AUC. There are no adequate and well-controlled studies of sildenafil in pregnant women.

Geriatric Use: Healthy elderly volunteers (65 years or over) had a reduced clearance of sildenafil (see **CLINICAL PHARMACOLOGY: Pharmacokinetics in Special Populations**). Since higher plasma levels may increase both the efficacy and incidence of adverse events, a starting dose of 25 mg should be considered (see **DOSAGE and ADMINISTRATION**).

ADVERSE REACTIONS

PRE-MARKETING EXPERIENCE:
VIAGRA was administered to over 3700 patients (aged 19-87 years) during clinical trials worldwide. Over 550 patients were treated for longer than one year.

In placebo-controlled clinical studies, the discontinuation rate due to adverse events for VIAGRA (2.5%) was not significantly different from placebo (2.3%). The adverse events were generally transient and mild to moderate in nature.

In trials of all designs, adverse events reported by patients receiving VIAGRA were generally similar. In fixed-dose studies, the incidence of some adverse events increased with dose. The nature of the adverse events in flexible-dose studies, which more closely reflect the recommended dosage regimen, was similar to that for fixed-dose studies.

When VIAGRA was taken as recommended (on an as-needed basis) in flexible-dose, placebo-controlled clinical trials, the following adverse events were reported:

TABLE 2. ADVERSE EVENTS REPORTED BY
≥2% OF PATIENTS TREATED WITH VIAGRA AND MORE FREQUENT ON DRUG THAN PLACEBO
IN PRN FLEXIBLE-DOSE
PHASE II/III STUDIES

Adverse Event	Percentage of Patients VIAGRA N=734	Reporting Event PLACEBO N=725
Headache	16%	4%
Flushing	10%	1%
Dyspepsia	7%	2%
Nasal Congestion	4%	2%
Urinary Tract Infection	3%	2%
Abnormal Vision¹	3%	0%
Diarrhea	3%	1%
Dizziness	2%	1%
Rash	2%	1%

¹Abnormal Vision: Mild and transient, predominantly color tinge to vision, but also increased sensitivity to light or blurred vision. In these studies, only one patient discontinued due to abnormal vision.

Other adverse reactions occurred at a rate of >2%, but equally common on placebo: respiratory tract infection, back pain, flu syndrome, and arthralgia.

In fixed-dose studies, dyspepsia (17%) and abnormal vision (11%) were more common at 100 mg than at lower doses. At doses above the recommended dose range, adverse events were similar to those detailed above but generally were reported more frequently.

The following events occurred in < 2% of patients in controlled clinical trials; a causal relationship to VIAGRA is uncertain. Reported events include those with a plausible relation to drug use; omitted are minor events and reports too imprecise to be meaningful:

Body as a whole: face edema, photosensitivity reaction, shock, asthenia, pain, chills, accidental fall, abdominal pain, allergic reaction, chest pain, accidental injury.

Cardiovascular: angina pectoris, AV block, migraine, syncope, tachycardia, palpitation, hypotension, postural hypotension, myocardial ischemia, cerebral thrombosis, cardiac arrest, heart failure, abnormal electrocardiogram, cardiomyopathy.

Digestive: vomiting, glossitis, colitis, dysphagia, gastritis, gastroenteritis, esophagitis, stomatitis, dry mouth, liver function tests abnormal, rectal hemorrhage, gingivitis.

Hemic and Lymphatic: anemia and leukopenia.

Metabolic and Nutritional: thirst, edema, gout, unstable diabetes, hyperglycemia, peripheral edema, hyperuricemia, hypoglycemic reaction, hypernatremia.

Musculoskeletal: arthritis, arthrosis, myalgia, tendon rupture, tenosynovitis, bone pain, myasthenia, synovitis.

Nervous: ataxia, hypertonia, neuralgia, neuropathy, paresthesia, tremor, vertigo, depression, insomnia, somnolence, abnormal dreams, reflexes decreased, hypesthesia.

Respiratory: asthma, dyspnea, laryngitis, pharyngitis, sinusitis, bronchitis, sputum increased, cough increased.

Skin and Appendages: urticaria, herpes simplex, pruritus, sweating, skin ulcer, contact dermatitis, exfoliative dermatitis.

Special Senses: mydriasis, conjunctivitis, photophobia, tinnitus, eye pain, deafness, ear pain, eye hemorrhage, cataract, dry eyes.

Urogenital: cystitis, nocturia, urinary frequency, breast enlargement, urinary incontinence, abnormal ejaculation, genital edema and anorgasmia.

POST-MARKETING EXPERIENCE:
Cardiovascular
Serious cardiovascular events, including myocardial infarction, sudden cardiac death, ventricular arrhythmia, cerebrovascular hemorrhage, transient ischemic attack and hypertension, have been reported post-marketing in temporal association with the use of VIAGRA. Most, but not all, of these patients had preexisting cardiovascular risk factors. Many of these events were reported to occur during or shortly after sexual activity, and a few were reported to occur shortly after the use of VIAGRA without sexual activity. Others were reported to have occurred hours to days after the use of VIAGRA

and sexual activity. It is not possible to determine whether these events are related directly to VIAGRA, to sexual activity, to the patient's underlying cardiovascular disease, to a combination of these factors, or to other factors (see **WARNINGS** for further important cardiovascular information).

Other events
Other events reported post-marketing to have been observed in temporal association with VIAGRA and not listed in the pre-marketing adverse reactions section above include:

Nervous: seizure and anxiety.

Urogenital: prolonged erection, priapism (see **WARNINGS**) and hematuria.

Ocular: diplopia, temporary vision loss/decreased vision, ocular redness or bloodshot appearance, ocular burning, ocular swelling/pressure, increased intraocular pressure, retinal vascular disease or bleeding, vitreous detachment/traction and paramacular edema.

OVERDOSAGE

In studies with healthy volunteers of single doses up to 800 mg, adverse events were similar to those seen at lower doses but incidence rates were increased.

In cases of overdose, standard supportive measures should be adopted as required. Renal dialysis is not expected to accelerate clearance as sildenafil is highly bound to plasma proteins and it is not eliminated in the urine.

DOSAGE AND ADMINISTRATION

For most patients, the recommended dose is 50 mg taken, as needed, approximately 1 hour before sexual activity. However, VIAGRA may be taken anywhere from 4 hours to 0.5 hour before sexual activity. Based on effectiveness and toleration, the dose may be increased to a maximum recommended dose of 100 mg or decreased to 25 mg. The maximum recommended dosing frequency is once per day.

The following factors are associated with increased plasma levels of sildenafil: age >65 (40% increase in AUC), hepatic impairment (e.g., cirrhosis, 80%), severe renal impairment (creatinine clearance <30 mL/min, 100%), and concomitant use of potent cytochrome P450 3A4 inhibitors [ketoconazole, itraconazole, erythromycin (182%), saquinavir (210%)]. Since higher plasma levels may increase both the efficacy and incidence of adverse events, a starting dose of 25 mg of VIAGRA in these patients.

Ritonavir greatly increased the systemic level of sildenafil in a study of healthy, non-HIV infected volunteers (11-fold increase in AUC, see **Drug Interactions**.) Based on these pharmacokinetic data, it is recommended not to exceed a maximum single dose of 25 mg of VIAGRA in a 48 hour period.

VIAGRA was shown to potentiate the hypotensive effects of nitrates and its administration in patients who use nitric oxide donors or nitrates in any form is therefore contraindicated.

HOW SUPPLIED

VIAGRA® (sildenafil citrate) is supplied as blue, film-coated, rounded-diamond-shaped tablets containing sildenafil citrate equivalent to the nominally indicated amount of sildenafil as follows:

	25 mg	50 mg	100 mg
Obverse	VGR25	VGR50	VGR100
Reverse	PFIZER	PFIZER	PFIZER
Bottle of 30	NDC-0069-4200-30	NDC-0069-4210-30	NDC-0069-4220-30
Bottle of 100	N/A	NDC-0069-4210-66	NDC-0069-4220-66

Recommended Storage: Store at controlled room temperature, 15° to 30°C (59° to 86°F).

R_x only

© 2000 PFIZER INC

Printed in U.S.A.
Revised Jan. 2000